PLEASE LEAVE THE LIGHTS ON:

An Incredible Story of Recovering from Traumatic Brain Injury

Harold Holder

With Bill M. West

PLEASE LEAVE THE LIGHTS ON:

AN INCREDIBLE STORY OF RECOVERING FROM TRAUMATIC BRAIN INJURY

Harold Holder

Copyright © 2011 by Harold Holder

All rights reserved.

This publication is protected under the US Copyright Act of 1976 and all other applicable international, federal, state and local laws, and all rights are reserved.

No part of this publication may be reproduced without the prior written permission of the publisher and the author, except for brief passages in connection with a review. Requests for reproduction should be addressed to:

GhostWest, LLC 510 E. Plumb Lane Ste. A Reno, Nevada 89502.

Email: BMW@GhostWest.com.

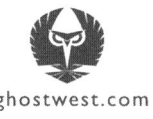

ghostwest.com

Compiled and Formatted by: GhostWest, LLC

ISBN: 1466405597

EAN-13: 978-1466405592

Printed in the United States of America

Dedication

I dedicate this humble effort to my beautiful wife, Anna Maria, who courageously and selflessly, spoon-fed me literally, figuratively and mentally through the black stormy uncertain ordeal we faced as a family. She did it with grace and poise. And to my young son Charlie, who, with maturity beyond his age of 5, faced the possible loss of his father bravely. His regular post surgery visits with his big brown eyes and smiling face were strong motivations to get on a fast track for recovery. Each visit was positive and full of encouragement. My number one son, Hal, Jr., took the walk with me to the pre-op room giving me as much reassurances as he could and retained his creditability, faced with the fresh facts he had from the surgeon. He filled the visit voids with all kinds of odd hour visits, giving me realistic and down-to-earth updates on the outside forces we were facing from people who were planning to take our company from us.

Acknowledgments

With sincere appreciation, I wish to acknowledge the gifted neurosurgeon Doctor Jay K. Morgan of The Sierra Neurosurgery Group. He expertly diagnosed my situation quickly, gave me my options (none) and proceeded to use his God-given talents to produce a result considerably north (better than) of his initial professional assessment. And to Doctor Richard H. Bryan, Jr., who instructed the fast action for the emergency room at Renown South Meadows, which resulted in the examination, findings, CAT scan and delivery of my case to Doctor Morgan. As a friend, Dr. Bryan did all this while on a road trip in California after getting an early morning panic call, on his personal cell phone, from my wife Anna. And to the outstanding professional staff and executives of the Renown Regional Medical Center, Reno. I wish to add, they were beyond excellent. To the therapy specialists—again, thank you. I attempted to highlight their importance in the body of the book. All the acknowledgments are, I am sure, understated, but are most heartfelt and sincere.

Table of Contents

Dedication iii
Acknowledgments v
Chapter 1   Wake Up Dying 1
Chapter 2   Odds of Living: 50/50 5
Chapter 3   Developing A Silent Faceless
             Monster Within 9
Chapter 4   The First 96 Hours 13
Chapter 5   Who I Am 19
Chapter 6   Jogging My Memory 27
Chapter 7   Running My Mind 31
Chapter 8   Merit Badges 35
Chapter 9   Learning to Fly 39
Chapter 10   Abilities Rediscovered 45
Chapter 11   Something to Say 51
Chapter 12   Actions Speak Louder
             Than Words 53
Chapter 13   A Home Built With Milestones 59
Chapter 14   Taking Chances 69
Chapter 15   Picking Up The Pace 75
Chapter 16   Business as Unusual 81
Chapter 17   The Slow Process 87
Chapter 18   Observations From The Editor 99
Accompanying Photographs 105
Epilogue 113

Chapter 1

Wake Up Dying

On November 13th, 2008 I awoke in the middle of the night only to stumble out of my bed and crumble to the floor. I was having an impossible time controlling my legs. It was a phenomenon I had never experienced. The loss of coordination concerned me enough to allow my wife, Anna, to drive me to the hospital; even though I insisted we wait until morning. Because I had recently been sick on and off, which was rare for me, my doctors had previously misdiagnosed my illness as bacterial pneumonia.

However, when Anna called my cardiologist, Dr. Richard Bryan, he strongly suggested that I complete a CAT scan as soon as possible. When Anna explained my coordination struggles, Dr. Bryan believed there could be something going on with me neurologically. He phoned doctors that he trusted and arranged for me to have a CAT scan that morning. When the results came back I inquired if everything was in order. I vividly remember the technician's response: "There's something serious going on here." As I heard those words, disbelief. In spite of my pilot training that emphasized trust in your instruments, I still had a flash of hope for the possibility of false or flawed test results. If that were not the case, how bad was it? I was searching for something—anything—that would lessen the trouble I was facing; my efforts proved to be fruitless.

After seeing the CAT scan image it was clear that someone with no medical experience could have diagnosed the problem. In fact, the doctor commented, "Even a janitor could have diagnosed the problem." A significant amount of blood was clotting in a confined space and putting pressure on my brain, which was the reason I was having trouble with my motor skills.

The seriousness set in along with the anxiety as I was being prepped for surgery. The doctors said they needed to operate immediately. I remember trying to catch my thoughts as Anna left to pull our son, Charlie, from school. I was not ready to tell anyone goodbye, let alone my five-year-old son.

My time in the Marine Corps branded into me not to fear death. I remembered the iconic saying, "Cowards die a thousand deaths, the brave die but once." Still attempting to have some control over the situation as I was being rolled into surgery, I told the neurosurgeon, Dr. Jay Morgan, "I am going into this with a 155 IQ and I would like to come out with the same."

He replied, "I'll do my best." Reality time.

Although surgery itself is always a serious measure, especially when you are rushed into it like I had been, I did not fully understand how critical my condition was. I do not remember the operating room or counting backwards or any of those scenes that precede an operation. All I remember was uncertainty. Then black.

Chapter 2

Odds of Living: 50/50

The injury I suffered is known in the medical world as a hematoma, which means an accumulation of blood. My variety was complicated subdural, meaning the blood was gathering between my brain and the dura, which is the tough lining that surrounds the brain. The distinction is because there is also a condition called an epidural hematoma in which the blood pools between the skull and the dura. Neither variety is preferred over the other as both epidural and subdural hematomas are serious head traumas. Subdural hematomas occur in only 15 percent of head injuries. Of those 15 percent, one in five prove to be fatal. However, since my condition was diagnosed as a "complicated" subdural hematoma, my chances of living were even slimmer; around 50 percent of patients whose injuries are labeled "complicated" die.

While head injuries are common, about 1.5 million in the United States annually, complicated subdural hematomas only occur in approximately 2 percent of patients suffering from head injuries. Many surgeons consider complicated subdural hematomas to be the most serious of head injuries because they often require prompt diagnosis and immediate surgical intervention. While the injury is more frequent in males, with a male-to-female ratio of 4:1, they are rare in older adults because the dura matter has formed tightly to the skullcap. However, in my situation the hematoma was able to find an area to clot and cause serious complication.

Four months after my surgery the country's awareness of severe head injuries skyrocketed when the young talented actress Natasha Richardson died two days after a minor skiing accident. When I read what the autopsy, on March 19th, 2009, revealed, it was sobering: Richardson had died from a hematoma, only hers was epidural. She had been skiing on a beginner's hill in Northeastern Canada when she took a mild fall. She was not wearing a helmet. She declined medical attention and went back to her hotel room complaining of a headache. An hour later she took an ambulance to a nearby hospital. Twenty-four hours later she flew back to a New York hospital. Twenty-four hours after arrival she was dead. Richardson was 45. The autopsy suggested that when Richardson fell, she hit her head and tore an artery inside of her skull. Since her initial symptoms were so subtle, doctors did not press the need for surgery, which would have relieved the pressure off her brain and most likely saved her life.

When blood inside the skull gathers, it has nowhere to push besides on the brain. The skull itself cannot expand. Since there is little open space inside the skull, it does not take a large amount of blood to produce a great deal of pressure on the brain. As little as three ounces of blood can be life threatening. According to a New York Times article about Richardson's fatal injury, "As a general rule, doctors say that any head injury should be treated within the so-called golden hour after it occurs."[i] Unfortunately, Richardson's brain was not seriously looked at within that "golden" hour, as is the case with many seemingly mild blows to the head.

If a neurosurgeon can diagnose the condition promptly, usually by way of a CAT scan, then the chances of them being able to relieve the brain pressure are good. Neurosurgeons treat the injury by cutting out a part of the skull to drain the built-up fluid, as they did in my situation. For Richardson, her hematoma developed quickly and proved to be fatal. For me, the bleeding was much, much slower—probably over a period of years.

---

[i] See http://www.time.com/time/magazine/article/0,9171,1887856,00.html

Chapter 3

Developing A Silent Faceless Monster Within

One month before the operation I had gotten dizzy, slipped and hit my cheek at the bottom of the staircase in our home. One year before the operation I had started to periodically get sick, which has always been rare for me. Six years before the operation I slipped on a patch of ice, knocked myself unconscious and awoke freezing and alone in the middle of my snowy driveway. All of these occurrences could have played a part in what eventually became blood seepage in my skull. However, it is impossible to determine with certainty which of the happenings helped develop the bleeding and which resulted because of it.

On a particularly cold and snowy morning in January of 2004, I was walking down our steep, winding driveway while Anna and Charlie were visiting Anna's sister in New Jersey. Without warning I slipped on a patch of ice and bounced the back of my head off the frozen asphalt. The fall knocked me out cold. When I came to, I knew the impact could have potentially done damage and I decided to go to the hospital. As is normal procedure when dealing with blunt head injuries, the doctors ran a CAT scan. The results showed nothing to be alarmed about. However, substantial swelling could have been inhibiting the bleeding. Only when the inflammation subsided would a CAT scan have been able to reveal the monster that I had awakened.

One year before the operation I started getting sick more frequently than any other time in my life. Like any child his age, my son Charlie often comes down with minor colds, sniffles and infections. However, I rarely come down with any symptoms. I attributed my periodic illnesses with the intense amount of stress that I was carrying because of work. As I will explain in more detail later in this book, a financial hailstorm had obliterated my company and I was working long hours in an attempt to keep it above water.

One month before the operation I bruised my cheek when I fell at the bottom of the stairs after momentarily blacking out. Anna called 9-1-1 and an ambulance soon arrived to take me to a local hospital. The doctors ran a serious of tests, did some blood work and diagnosed me with bacterial pneumonia. The diagnosis lined up because of my frequent illnesses, spotty coordination, the weakness I had been experiencing and the blackout that likely was the result of a sporadic drop in blood pressure. The doctors put me on intravenous antibiotics and kept me over night. They did not run a CAT scan.

For the entire month between the bacterial-pneumonia diagnosis and my brain surgery, I continued to feel weak and ill. My health, which was usually not an issue, was well below my normal and it was draining me physically. I knew something was wrong, but I believed the diagnosis to be accurate and thought it was taking an extended period of time for me to recover from the pneumonia.

Ten hours before I would be red lined into surgery, I found myself struggling in the dark to get back into my bed at home. The disturbance awakened Anna and she knew something was wrong. My coordination was off, way off. My legs were numb and half of my body felt asleep. We were both worried, but because everything else felt normal, I insisted that we wait until morning to call Dr. Bryan, who had been a longtime friend as well as my cardiologist.

Eight hours before my surgery I was back at the hospital and looking to a CAT scan for answers.

Three hours before my surgery I was reviewing the results with Dr. Jay Morgan; something was serious.

Two hours before my surgery I was having what could prove to be my last conversations with my five-year-old son and beautiful wife.

At 5:30 p.m., my day at the hospital was reaching its climax. I was prepped and wheeled back for a dangerous brain operation, unsure if I would ever recover. No matter how long it takes for subdural hematomas to demand attention, they all lead to the same fork in the road: Surgery or death.

Chapter 4

The First 96 Hours

I woke up on what I would later learn was mid-morning on November 14th, 2008. My thinking was fuzzy, cluttered and remained polluted with uncertainty. I began to understand pieces of the puzzle I was in and I attempted to compile a self-assessment. I was able to put together that I had survived the brain surgery—even though I was unsure if the operation had taken an hour, a half day or even longer.

I recognized that I was restrained. This did not immediately strike me as necessary since the only movement I had was in my eyes. But, as I took in more of my surroundings I noticed the array of tubes intertwined with various sensitive areas of my body, mostly my head. I was restrained because I was a threat to myself. A lengthy scar now fish-hooked from the top center of my skull around to the back of my right ear—splitting my skull into two vastly different terrains. The landscape to the right of the hook was a battlefield—shaved to the skull, bruised and beet-colored. The section to the left of the scar was unmolested, albeit patchy with uneven stubble, which was hardly a pressing concern at this point.

Now, nearly 77 years after my soft spot as an infant had formed and closed, I again had a fragile section on the top of my skull. Only this time it was the size of a meat hook and was held together with 39 metal staples.

 The medical team had fixed a drain to my skull to act as a trench in which excess fluid could flow and collect in a small plastic container. Uneducated on the condition in which one should emerge from an intrusive brain surgery, I was confused if all of the equipment I was joined with equaled a success or not. I knew I had survived, but how much of me? The fluids cycling through my body, the consistent beeps of various machines, the restraints and the skull drain all suggested to me that I was in a fragile state. After all, a mere staple puller could have spilled my brain to the floor.

 I sought some small form of encouragement and I found it through my ability to work my brain. As I fought through the fuzz caused by all the drugs in my system, I remembered a quote from one of my favorite authors, Ernest Hemingway: "My brain is my capital." I started to test my brain capital by remembering simple occurrences: *I had survived brain surgery. I was atop a hospital bed. I could identify a wall, a door, the ceiling.* It only took a matter of minutes before a number of dark thoughts worked their way through my mind: *Would I ever regain the strength to get myself out of this bed? Would I ever walk again? Is this the bed/room/hospital in which I will die?* I thought of my 93-year-old mother. Would I ever see her again or enjoy another conversation with someone whom I thought was so wise and insightful? As quickly as these impossible-to-answer questions weaved their way into my mind, I crushed them and concentrated on the present.

My lucidity allowed me to understand more about my surroundings. To my relief, Anna was standing brave and beautiful beside my bed. Our son Charlie was by her side, handsome and strong. My other son, Hal Jr., had visited me before my last pre-operation talk with Dr. Morgan. While I did not want to concern Anna and young Charlie, I could be direct with Hal Jr. and express my concerns surrounding the surgery. Later I would learn that Dr. Morgan spoke with Anna prior to my surgery and Anna had bravely taken the brunt of the seriousness of my circumstances. Dr. Morgan had prepped her for the operation and she knew the odds of my survival were far less than favorable. Thankfully, while she is much younger than I, she has always demonstrated a higher level of maturity.

I began to think about the family members in my presence. Charlie had courageously came with Anna and I thought how he must have been as confused as I was about who was sprawled across the hospital bed in the Intensive Care Unit of Renown Medical Center. I hoped he was not considering the possibilities of my state being permanent, for he needed much more from his father.

I knew it was necessary to think of the more positive aspects of waking up. Alive. My current mindset would dictate my progress and help lead me the rest of the way. These were the infant stages of recovery. I aimed at staying positive by remembering how great of a blessing it was to survive such a serious surgery.

At this point, at least to my knowledge, I had not yet seen Dr. Morgan. Instead of being consumed by the fear that this would be the first in a series of complicated surgeries, I hoped he had achieved the results he desired. With each thought I was conditioning myself to stay positive. There were far too many worries surrounding my situation. It was, to make a severe understatement, overwhelming.

I remembered a book by Eugene O'Kelly titled *Chasing Daylight* in which the author was given three months to live after being diagnosed with inoperable brain tumors. Somehow, O'Kelly's outlook was surprisingly uplifting. He considered it a blessing to have a doctor administer a timetable that estimated how long he had before his life expired. O'Kelly used the time he had to become more focused on the present and adequately unwind all of the meaningful relationships in his life. Towards the beginning of his book, O'Kelly states:

> *Because of the factors surrounding my dying—my relative youth, my continued possession of mental facility and otherwise good physical health, my freedom from daily pain, and the proximity of loved ones, most of whom were themselves still in their prime—I took a different approach to my last*

100 days, one that required that I keep my eyes as wide open as possible. Even with blurry vision.

O'Kelly's optimism was empowering, even as I lay physically powerless on a hospital bed in the heart of the ICU.

Chapter 5

Who I am

When most authors give their biography, they tend to start at their roots and pick up pieces of their identity along the way. While this is a story of my brain injury and ensuing recovery rather than an autobiography, a full and detailed bio is not necessary; so I will be brief. I was born in Anniston, Alabama on June 25th, 1931 and I spent the majority of my childhood in Pensacola, Florida. Despite my family living the definitive poor lifestyle, I never considered myself *poor*. Living in a house with no plumbing and selling scrap metal out of my wagon at age five, I learned to work with what I had, which was very little. At the time, the world was preparing to go to war for the second time and metal scraps were in demand for recycling into munitions. On most nights, the change I collected from the bits of iron determined whether or not my family had dinner on the table.

From a very early age, I always kept busy and pushed forward. To contribute what I could to my family, I worked the kinds of odd jobs that would spark a child-labor lawsuit today. Back then, however, it was just something that needed to be done.

After gaining a fairly typical high school education, I joined the Marines. My mother used to say that I joined the Marines not in search of discipline, but because I was disciplined. I deeply connected to the Marine code of life and to this day I identify myself as a Marine. I suppose it is similar to being an Olympian: Once you compete in the Olympics, you are forever an Olympian. Once you join the Corps, you are forever a Marine.

As I mentioned earlier, I believe I started my business career at five years old when I was selling scraps of metal on the back streets of Pensacola. My formal business career, however, started with Sears, Roebuck & Company after I served in the Marines. In my 15 years with Sears, I had 14 different titles including Director of Sales Promotion for the entire South. I never doubted that I could run Sears, but I hit a ceiling in the company because of its strict "rule" that forbid anyone from becoming an officer before their 50th birthday. Not willing to sit around until my age caught up with Sears' ageist policy, I left the organization in 1969. That same year I became the president of a company that was listed on the New York Stock Exchange: Cunningham Drug Stores based in Detroit, Michigan.

While I believed it was an honor to become president of a publicly traded company, I joined Cunningham when it was faltering and spiraling downward. However, in dealing with what I had, I returned the company to profitability after only 18 months. In doing so, I established what would be my *modus operandi* for the rest of my business career: Capturing failing companies and returning them to success.

Twelve months into my stint as president of Cunningham Drug Stores, I made my first million dollars. I remember my accountant calling me on a late Friday afternoon to congratulate me. He described how he had just totaled my personal balance sheet, which had broken the million-dollar mark for the first time and was moving upward. When I hung up the phone, I returned to the deck of my home in Bloomfield Hills, Michigan and finished cooking family hamburgers as part of our normal routine. Early the next day I remained on task with my normal weekly routine: I cleaned and organized the garage. Looking back on this bit of financial news, it was truly a non-event, and I treated it as such.

Two years after joining Cunningham, I left in order to take over as president of Rahall Communications, a troubled cluster of radio and TV outlets based in St. Petersburg, Florida. After 18 months of dedicated work with Rahall, I had another 18-month turnaround from loss to profit and this helped to solidify my place in the business world. Financially battered companies were requesting for me to take over their firms and return them to profitability. In 1973, two years after first taking over Rahall Communications, I left my position and agreed to join American Agronomics. The company, which was a big player in the orange business, had recently been beaten and bruised by several lawsuits and an investigation by the Securities and Exchange Commission (SEC). American Agronomics had a surplus of land and I quickly sold off any of it that was not fit for supporting orange groves. After trimming the fat and injecting the company with my own money, I had a strong foundation on which to re-grow the business.

Business media began focusing on my ability to rescue large companies and started publically referring to me as a "turnaround artist." A feature in Fortune Magazine stated that when I arrived as president and chief executive at American Agronomics,

> …*the company was in desperate straits. Its reputation was shattered and no one was willing to buy its orange groves. It was laden with debt from its purchase of the properties, and was losing money. It seemed doomed. But liquidation didn't suit Holder's plans or his temperament.*[ii]

In the mid-1970s, I was honored to be a personal subject in a case study on turnaround and reconstruction ability produced by the Harvard School of Business. In 1975 I published my first book, *Don't Shoot! I'm Only a Trainee*, which notable businesses such as General Motors used as their training tool for new hires. The original run of my first book was 4,000 with a selling price of $4.95. A recent visit to Amazon.com pulled up a listing for an autographed copy of *Don't Shoot* priced at $299.95. My original compensation for writing the book was $1 per copy,

---

[ii]Louis, A. M. (1981, January 26). Squeezing Gold. *Fortune*, 78–82.

which was nothing to scoff at for creating a book I thoroughly enjoyed writing. A lifetime of writing notes, essays and material for several other books are in safekeeping. Now, since I have been blessed to continue living, I plan on finishing all of them.

In the early 1980s, my career was moving in the right direction. American Agronomics had a glowing financial future as I continued to expand it, which caused earnings to continue to rise each year. American Agronomics had three main orange groves, including the Joshua Grove, which was roughly the size of San Francisco and the largest contiguous orange grove in the world at the time. After returning American Agronomics to profitability by way of prolific orange groves, an act of God nearly wiped out our biggest moneymaker. An article titled *Turnaround Artist* in an issue of *Florida Business* summed it up best:

> *On January 12, 1982, American Agronomics lost $65 million in 24 hours when Florida was hit by the worst freeze in a hundred years. When he saw the damage to the orange trees, Holder says he felt a little like Scarlett O-Hara in Gone With the Wind when she dug a turnip out of the ground and said "I promise never to be hungry again."*[iii]

[iii]Crews, L. (1986, February). Harold Holder. *Florida Business/ Tampa Bay*, 28–31.

Becoming so dependent on a resource that could be devastated by a turn in the weather was an enormous business mistake and American Agronomics was lucky to live through it. I promised myself to never let that happen again and I worked diligently to create revenue streams that were not reliant on oranges. The first two years after the freeze, American Agronomics lost money. But, in the third year, we returned to profitability and had significantly diversified as a company.

In 1987 I stepped away from American Agronomics. That same year, stockholders voted to change the company's name to Orange-co Inc. I sold off most of my stock and agreed to become a paid consultant for the next 24 months. I became managing director of The Holder Group, Inc., which invested in and owned a variety of private companies.

In 1999 I moved west to Reno, Nevada when The Holder Group purchased the Sundance Casino in Winnemucca, Nevada—marking my entrance into the gaming industry. Later that year, The Holder Group purchased nearly 95% of the common stock of Summit Casinos-Nevada Inc., which owned The Silver Club Hotel/Casino in Sparks, Nevada and the El Capitan Lodge and Casino in Hawthorne, Nevada.

As I will explain in further detail in Chapter 16, *Business as Unusual*, The Holder Group was seriously challenged during the time surrounding my brain surgery. Throughout my lengthy and varied business career I have encountered more than my fair share of obstacles. I have also dealt with some of the most astringent of adversaries. However, none ever proved to be as callus as those who threatened my business while a traumatic brain injury threatened my life.

Chapter 6

Jogging My Memory

Restrained and stretched out across a hospital bed in Renown Medical's ICU, I used the one tool that was available to me: My memory. As long as I was confined to this hospital room, in this hospital bed, I would jog my memory and build my mental strength. Although at this point I could not lift a paper clip, I could lift my spirits by thinking back to some of my most precious memories. I immediately went to the most cherished experience I have: Marrying my beautiful Anna Maria. While remembering our wedding I could work through my memory to find the dates, locations and conditions to piece together all of the special moments that surrounded the event.

December 17th, 1996—I knew the date of our wedding with cunning precision and certainty. I remembered the date with such conviction that I was encouraged to branch out to other details. Anna and I exchanged vows in Athens, Greece. We stood in close proximity to the Parthenon on the Acropolis (a crowning hill overlooking the brilliant city of Athens). Months earlier I had arranged with the manager at the Hotel Grande Bretagne to book the top-floor corner suite, which overlooked the center of Athens. At night, we could look out our windows and see the Parthenon with spectacular lights illuminating the site. The view stole the air from our lungs nightly.

We were in Athens for days waiting for sweeping rains to clear from the city. The storms were relentless, but we would be damned if it was going to rain on our wedding day. When we awoke on the morning of December 17th, 1996, sunlight poured through the windows of our hotel and filled every corner of our suite. Consumed by excitement, Anna began to prepare our wedding attire. She had her hair beautifully prepared at a salon near our hotel. Remembering the events that surrounded our wedding gave me inspiration to put the details in order and create a clearer perspective.

We hired a driver/bodyguard named Nicholas to navigate through the streets, language barriers and other complications of getting us onto the Acropolis, which was filled with suspicious Greek security guards. Nicholas was an understanding and very capable young man. He had a take-charge attitude that allowed Anna and me to enjoy each other's company without stressing over minor obstacles.

Before we met Nicholas, we had a bump in our trip that nearly derailed us completely. The airline had lost the suitcase in which Anna had painstakingly packed her wedding dress. I remembered the tears that rolled down Anna's face at the Athens International Airport when she thought her dress had been misplaced forever. However, the next day an airport representative delivered the missing piece of luggage to our hotel. Anna immediately placed the suitcase on our bed and pulled out the most beautiful pale-yellow dress. She had designed it herself and had the piece tailored by a seamstress in Tampa Bay. To be modest, her gown was stunning, which fit the occasion on the most important day in both of our lives.

Chapter 7

Running My Mind

As I thought about our wedding, I remembered why the Hotel Grande Bretagne had such a special meaning to us. Two years prior to our wedding we had stayed at the Hotel Grande Bretagne when I was registered to run in a marathon that covered the original route of the first marathon. I had looked forward to this historic race since I had started my running career when I was 57, nearly five years prior.

I was inspired to begin a steady running regiment after visiting the Pritikin Longevity Center on the Pacific Ocean in Santa Monica, California. I originally traveled to Pritikin to take a self-assessment of my life. During my stay I came to understand the value that the staff put on walking as a beneficial form of exercise—one that people can practice their entire lives. I had found motivation and inspiration at Pritikin and gravitated towards running because I could get twice the amount of exercise than I could while walking. After months of sticking to a steady running program when I got back to my home in Florida, I decided to enter my first five-kilometer race. I had set a personal goal and I was dedicated to making a strong showing in my first official race; really I just wanted to finish and not embarrass myself.

Over the first few years after I began running, I completed a number of 5ks and 10ks in the Tampa Bay area; they were all extremely satisfying. I was prolific in entering races and to date I have accumulated over 300 plaques, awards, ribbons, trophies and certificates; all for ranking within my age group at various races. In 1989 I entered to be selected to run in the New York Marathon. Because of its popularity, the first 8,000 entrants were accepted and the remaining participants were selected in a lottery fashion. An investment banker friend of mine in New York hand carried my registration form to the entry office as soon as it opened. This ensured I would get a bib number to run in one of the most celebrated marathons in the world.

The 26.2 miles of a marathon make for a pretty anti-climactic event considering the amount of training that is required. Running demands strict discipline. For each marathon I would train a minimum of 12 weeks and invest at least 750 miles to build my endurance. Anna was always extremely supportive in all of my running endeavors. Of the 15 marathons I have completed, she has been excitedly waiting at the finish line for 14 of them. I precisely remember the race in which Anna was absent and, through teasing, I have never let her live down the *one* she missed.

I was running in the Boston Marathon of 1991. The temperature at the start of the race was 42 degrees and it was raining lightly. By the end of the race, a large number of that year's 8,500 participants had fallen victim to hypothermia. Anna had stayed at the finish line for hours before returning to the hotel a few blocks away to warm her bones. The circumstances were dreary for runners and spectators alike and I certainly understood why Anna retreated to the warmth of the hotel room. But, to this day I still enjoy teasing her about missing me cross the finish line of just one of my 15 marathons.

These memories were precious to relive while lying immobile on the hospital bed. All of my running memories were so clear and I could get lost in them, replaying the details in my mind. I would later learn from Dr. Morgan and Dr. Bryan that my running played an important part in the beginning stages of my physical recovery. While confined to my hospital bed, I often relived the circumstances of the pinnacle of my running career: The Athens Marathon.

The Athens Marathon commemorates the trek of the soldier Pheidippides from the town of Marathon, Greece to Athens in 490 B.C. As the story has it, Pheidippides is said to have run the 40,000-meter route to bring news to Athens of a Greek victory over the Persians. Nearly 2,400 years later, in 1896, Athens hosted the first modern Olympic Games and 25 runners covered Phedippides' route in what would become the modern marathon. Only nine runners finished the race and eight of them were Greek. The marathon was the last scheduled event of the 1896 Games and the only contest to be won by a member of the host country.

The Athens Marathon in October of 1994 marked a tremendous milestone in my running career. Running over footprints on a road that was several thousand years old was extremely moving. The course started on a bridge in the city of Marathon, traveled the coastline north of Athens and ended in Athens at the first modern Olympic stadium. I remembered how emotional the race was and other details surrounding the event became sharp in my mind. My running career that had helped keep my physical fitness in check was now encouraging me mentally. I challenged myself to remember specifics from the Athens marathon. There were 1,500 entrants, 55 of them coming from America. I bonded with a number of the Americans and soon discovered they were all first timers in this epic race.

After the marathon, Anna and I retreated to the island of Mykonos so I could recover and relax. It was on one of the island's windy hills where I proposed to Anna. I was as elated to *remember* that she had said "yes" as I was 15 years ago when she actually had.

Chapter 8

Merit Badges

In the ICU, I constantly drifted in and out of conscious because of the heavy drug regiment the nurses were feeding me. When I was conscious I would drift in and out of special memories that I have had the good fortune to experience in my life. I also often thought about the little things I had left unfinished.

It was not the business or financial concerns that bothered me, but the personal responsibilities I had taken on before my surgery. For example, Charlie had been politely requesting (sometimes persisting) that I put on my Marine Corps dress blues for him. Months prior he had spotted them in my closet and his fascination kept him insisting that I sport them. When he would visit the hospital, I would look at his handsome face, into his big brown eyes, and think about his request that I had yet to fulfill. I regretted that prior to my surgery I had made excuses to get out of dragging my dress blues out of the closet. Now, it was all I could think about doing for Charlie and I prayed that one day soon I would be able to, before he lost interest.

Another personal responsibility that nagged its way through my mind was the thought of a birdhouse that sat uncompleted in my garage. I started building it for my lovely sister, Pat, but now it collected dust near my idle power tools. Not having control over my hands, I wondered if I would ever again be able to control the complex power tools that I so much enjoyed working with. Furthermore, I wondered if I would ever again possess the strength to manipulate even a flathead screwdriver. In all modesty, the birdhouse I was building was more than the delicate kind you might find for sale in the summer time at local craft shops. Because my sister had homes in central Florida and northeast Alabama, the birdhouse stood the chance of being decimated by hurricanes. The craftsmanship required to make a birdhouse hurricane-proof was time consuming, to say the least. But, the safety and comfort that would be afforded to a family of Alabama Yellowhammers or Florida Northern Mockingbirds was worth the tedious attention. I ached to get back to the birdhouse because I knew if I could finish it then I had once again regained the capability to handle the detailed craftsmanship.

I knew I was getting ahead of myself thinking about handling powerful skill saws and nail guns before I could even make a fist. I would first have to accomplish the miniscule tasks the ICU nurses were requesting of me. For example, on occasion a caretaker would place two fingers in the palm of my hand and ask me to squeeze. They were testing my dexterity, or, more appropriately, lack thereof. I was very self-conscious about being the piece of the puzzle that delayed the recovery process. Not being able to squeeze a nurse's fingers gave me the motivation to want to squeeze the hell out of them the next time such a request was made. After each finger squeeze that I demonstrated a pitiful performance, I would try and force my arms against the handrails of my bed, trying to get them to turn. I consciously made a decision to make this test a merit badge that I desperately wanted to earn; it would be the first of many. I knew if I earned this symbolic badge that I would be offered more opportunities on my path to recovery. The helplessness I felt is beyond description. Not being able to feed myself, use the toilet on my own or bathe without assistance was humbling, even borderline demoralizing. But, I thought, one merit badge at a time.

Soon, I was able to squeeze a nurse's fingers to the point she would have to ask me to stop. Even though I had no feeling in my hands, I still knew I was making progress. With this imaginary merit badge in my possession, I was able to move to my next, which came with a seductive reward. If I could reach up and work the gadget that was attached to my I.V., I would be allowed to administer morphine to myself intravenously. The contraption resembled a bicycle handlebar with a button in the middle that released morphine into my system, without the possibility of overdose. I was first able to reach the gadget with my right hand, and soon my left was capable as well. I was a switch hitter in the game of morphine allocation. While on the drug I realized that I could never again be critical of anyone who ever became addicted to morphine while in pain.

To me, it was the sweetest, purest condition-altering drug I had ever experienced. But, I was committed to remaining disciplined. I only administered morphine to myself when I felt the edge of pain creeping up, which, after recently having my skull split open, was every time the previous dose wore off.

Despite being in and out of a foggy drug stupor, I securely held onto my desire to exercise my mind. I was constantly either thinking positively about the present and future or struggling to remember important happenings of the past. I wanted to make every moment I was awake beneficial to my recovery process.

I am confident that I made a nuisance of myself in the eyes of the patient caretakers in the ICU. Because I did not want to pass out and wake up in a dark room, I reminded them daily to "please leave the lights on."

Chapter 9

Learning to Fly

I appreciated so much the warmth provided by the visits of those closest to me. Seeing Anna's smiling face and Charlie's soft expressions not only gave me something to look forward to each day, but also helped take the grimness out of my situation. To fill the visitor void when Anna and Charlie were not around, Hal Jr. would regularly come at odd times and keep me company. His visits were helpful to me because I felt I could be less guarded with my questions and self-evaluations. I appreciated the relaxed visiting hours the staff allowed. Anyone that has ever been in a situation similar to mine can attest to the priceless value of family visits. They always boosted my morale and provided pockets of certainty within the twilight zone of uncertainty in which I found myself.

On day four in the ICU, a speech pathologist paid me a visit. One of the first questions he asked me concerned my ability to identify directions on a compass rose. He asked me to tell him which way I would be heading if I was traveling north and made a 90-degree left turn. I quickly replied "west" and his smile indicated I had done something right. He was delighted I made my response so rapidly.

I believe I did so because I had been required to make instantaneous decisions countless times in all my years as an airplane pilot. More important than answering the specialist's question was the pleasure that thinking of my flying days brought me. It was another vast category of information that I could use to test my mental capacity.

In all my years of flying, I often told friends that I was not a good pilot; I was a *damn* good pilot. For as far back as I can remember, I have always truly loved to fly. For over 40 years I have been an active pilot. Since I bought my first airplane, a 175 Skylark single-engine Cessna, in 1968, there have been few periods in my life in which I did not own my own plane. Being a pilot always gave me motivation to stay physically fit and mentally astute. The thought of not being able to sit in the left seat of an aircraft and man the controls was very bitter to me. The visit from the speech pathologist opened a gratifying memory window into my flying days, but it also caused me to question if those days might all be behind me. Laying there thinking of flying had me remembering a poem I wrote more than 15 years earlier:

*The roll-out on the long
smooth runway
Throttles being pushed gently
forward all the way
The roll, the lift-off, the thrilling
climb
The excitement never wanes, even after
thousands of times.*

We knife through the black, windless,
still night
Engines purring softly without
sensation of flight
All indicators on the panel are friendly
and safely in the green
God, I love flying this machine.

With bright stars above us, my plane
and I
Are here together, trusting each other,
in our sky
Twinkling lights below; towns, villages
And once-in-a-while an airport beacon beams
Life is good, flying this machine.

The peace of this is very personal and
deep inside
A type of contentment requiring skill,
returning pride
A glance to instruments, all dials and
knobs, a check reassuring
This love may be hard for others to understand,
its fidelity so enduring.

Silence of voices now necessarily
broken,
To the assigned runway we descend
Instructions received, acknowledged, and
the plane glides gracefully toward the ground
Another flight almost at end.

*Smoothly we land, roll to slow
and taxi to the ramp
My thoughts, as the mixture goes to lean,
God, thank you for the gift to fly
this machine.*

The thought of never again being able to fly an airplane was not only too difficult for me to comprehend, but I was also getting ahead of myself, *again*. I could not allow myself to think about maneuvering a 10,000-pound aircraft 25,000 feet in the air when my ability to walk was still in question. I tried to compartmentalize these thoughts and forced myself to focus on the basics.

On my fifth day in the ICU, it was apparent to me that I was making progress in my recovery. Physically, my dexterity had increased and the nurses seemed pleased about the small gains in my motor skills. My speech was slowly improving, but I was still very deliberate in my word selection. I did not want anyone to be concerned about my slurring speech, which I knew was a natural occurrence after brain surgery. Mentally, my memory efforts were paying off by the hour. I did not need the input of a trained professional to know I was light years ahead of where I was when I first became conscious after surgery.

My determination to push hard for mental and physical recovery was growing with every waking moment. Yet, I received no indication as to how long I would remain in the ICU. I did know the staff was pushing for me to undergo occupational therapy and continued speech therapy in the near future. The very recommendation indicated the severity of my situation. After 96 hours in Intensive Care, the discussion concerning my move into a different unit of the hospital began. Progress, I hoped.

Chapter 10

Abilities Rediscovered

Five days off of the operating table and I was informed I would be relocated to the Rehabilitation Unit outside of the main Renown Medical Center. Before I was moved, I received a phone call from Dr. Bryan. He assured me he was following my progress and guaranteed that I would make a full recovery. I welcomed the warm words, but also slightly discounted his statement only because he was a dear friend and he knew encouragement could only help. I also had a surprising visit from the ER doctor who had misdiagnosed my condition as bacterial pneumonia one month earlier. He apologized to Anna for not probing deeper into my ailment and pushing for a CAT scan when I stayed overnight in the hospital after falling and hitting my cheek. I believe these doctors to be tremendous people and it is not in my nature to be critical of an immediate, albeit incorrect, diagnosis. It was very gentlemanly of him to communicate with Anna.

As I was prepped for the move, I was convinced that whatever was about to unfold could not possibly be as terrifying as my first few uncertain days in the ICU. Needless to say, I was pleased to see the ICU disappear behind me as I was rolled to the ambulance and driven to my next location.

When we arrived at the Rehabilitation Center, I was assigned to a two-bed hospital room and had the good fortune to occupy it alone for the first few days. I immediately recognized that my bed was located very close to the bathroom. I had developed a constant envy of people who could shower alone. However, the close proximity of the bathroom encouraged me that I could soon be one of those people if I continued to push toward physical improvement.

Within my first few days in the Rehabilitation Unit, I was visited by physical therapist Scott Peterson (not of the Scott and Laci Peterson court hearings). Scott communicated that he would like me to begin physical therapy in the next couple of days. Upon hearing the news I immediately inquired why we could not start the therapy right then. Obviously, since I had been lying in a bed the past five days, I was not preoccupied with other engagements. Scott replied with a number of responses: *I lacked proper clothing, I could not walk, my movement was limited.* Although his answers were appropriate, I did not accept his evaluation, which I felt was filled with less-than-important reasons. The only part of his response that I did not have immediate control over was my lack of "proper" clothing. "As far as the clothes are concerned," I said, "find me some I can use." I spoke with a tone that suggested I was not going to take "no" for an answer.

Scott went to the laundry room area in the occupational therapy facility and brought back a pair of four-sizes-too-large shorts and a used T-shirt. The clothes might have fit civilian-me, but hospital-me was down about 12 pounds. However, ill-fitting clothes were not going to delay me from beginning physical therapy. They slipped me into the clothes and strapped on a pair of running shoes that Anna had stored with my belongings. I was ready. Scott, along with the assistance of others, lowered me into a wheelchair, strapped me in and rolled me out of my new hospital room.

While swimming around inside someone else's clothes, I arrived at one of the two physical therapy gyms located at Renown's Rehabilitation Center. My first impression was heartbreaking. The physical therapists rolled me inside a room that seemed, upon first glance, to sprawl with activity. But, upon further review, each patient was diligently working at exercises that were very limited in activity. I saw a brain-injured teen struggling to learn to use a wheelchair. Across the room I watched a very attractive young lady work through a series of upper-body stretches—I was later told she would never walk again. They were aiming to strengthen her upper body so her muscle groups could be strong enough to give her mobility without the use of her legs. An assortment of people who were much younger than me filled the room.

The two physical therapy gyms can each accommodate up to 25 people at once—trainers and patients. On my first encounter there were, among others, stroke and heart attack victims, patients recovering from near-fatal car accidents and survivors of various brain injuries. I was reminded of a book by Alexander King called "Mine Enemy Grows Older" in which the author states, "I've seen the problem, and the problem is mine." I was frightened. Terrified. I thought *I don't belong here*, but in fact I did.

The main gym, which patients with brain injuries are initially kept out of because of the racket, is equipped with ramps, weights, a variety of workouts balls and wide blue stretching mats. The environment was filled with people doing very elementary activities. Some maneuvered down narrow walkways while clutching onto handrails. Others battled to roll light, inflated balls away from their bodies. One patient was focused on tossing a plastic ring onto a wooded peg four feet in front of him. A handful of people were stretching on soft gym mats with the assistance of physical therapists. After allowing my surroundings to soak in for a few minutes, I was curious how long these patients had been in therapy only to get to this point. I was certain they had made *some* degree of progress, but the big picture that was presented to me showed they were still struggling with basic foundational tasks. My immediate reaction was "this place is not for me." But, I was thinking in pre-surgery terms and knew I had to accept that my physical condition had somewhat deteriorated. I still could not help but think that I was better off than what I was witnessing. After all, mere weeks ago I was running for miles on my treadmill and maneuvering my three-ton Hummer across the interstate.

This first day of physical therapy amounted to little more than viewing the facilities. I was wheeled to the second gym, where I would be starting my physical therapy as part of what was called "acute inpatient rehab." This gym was quieter and a bit smaller. A gutted half automobile was located near the back wall. Patients would practice climbing in and out of the car to prove to the therapists that they could open a door, squat inside and return in one piece. Because this was the gym where patients with brain injuries started their therapy, all of the medical professionals had an understanding to keep the noise to a minimum. The collected whispers of encouragement made it that much more calm, but at the same time even that much more eerie.

My second day of physical therapy was more eventful. My first impression the day before had desensitized me to the environment and now I could focus on what I needed to do to kick-start my recovery. On this second day I had the pleasure of meeting Joe Volcskai, a talented physical therapist of 13 years who was as dedicated to my recovery as I was. Joe was interested in evaluating my condition so he could provide accurate treatment. My first impression of Joe was that he seemed very approachable. Before I was asked to make any movements, he took the time to tell me about himself. And, even though my speech was still slightly slurred, he gave me the chance to tell him what I could about myself.

I then showed Joe that I could make simple movements (e.g. get out of bed, stand up). I could move around without a walker, but Joe took note that my balance was off tremendously. I was unsteady. If I was asked to walk, turn around and return, I was at moderate risk of tumbling to the floor. As a precautionary measure, Joe recommended I used a walker for assistance. My attention and focus were fairly good, which he told me was rare with brain injuries. It was during this first assessment that I told Joe I was very motivated. With my speech as smooth as I could muster, I told him, "I am really determined to make a full recovery."

Chapter 11

Something to Say

After meeting with Joe for my first day of activity, I also met Sarah Roberts, SLP (Speech Language Pathologist), who would become my speech and occupational therapist. For the rest of my hospital stay, I would meet with Sarah twice per day, or once if I took on additional "home" work.

Sarah told me that the two main concerns with patients who suffered a severe brain injury were swallowing complications and communication and cognitive issues. Upon evaluation, Sarah and another speech pathologist determined that I was not having any problem swallowing. However, they did note that I was having mild cognitive difficulties that involved complex thinking skills such as planning, prioritizing and judgment. These cognitive skills that had come easy to me pre-surgery were now presenting a problem. After evaluation Sarah developed a mental-exercise regime that would help me regain complex thinking skills.

Sarah was very forthcoming with the seriousness of what I had been through. She provided me with very sobering evaluations of my surgery. She said if my brain again experienced blood pressure as high as it had been, it would cut off the blood supply to other brain cells and they would die. Sarah's information was enduring.

Long after my surgery I remember Dr. Morgan telling me that I had been "15 minutes away from dying." Even though his comments came well after the fact, I still reflect on how damn lucky I am. Anna told me that minutes after my surgery, Dr. Morgan had told her that he was encouraged because he had seen brain life and movement after the cavity of the hematoma had been cleared. But, even then, the degree of permanent damage could not be known for months or even years after the operation.

Sarah was very kind in educating me about brain injuries. Her vast knowledge sparked my continued interest to understand head injuries and the surgeries that aim to correct them.

During the first few days of physical and speech therapy, I was relieved to finally know what had been going on with me. Before the surgery I was having trouble walking, sometimes stumbling over. It felt as if I was experiencing mild vertigo but I could not put my finger on the problem. My motor skills were off and there was no explanation for it. Even though I was now much worse off than I had been pre-surgery, it was a relief to know that the problem had been pinpointed, addressed and, hopefully, corrected. While I still could not toss a ring onto a metal peg four feet in front of me, I was happy to know that a burden in my life was addressed and recovery was in my own control.

Chapter 12

Actions Speak Louder Than Words

Now faced with tedious physical therapy tasks, the next merit badge I was working toward was to become "room free." This meant I would be permitted to visit the toilet by myself, as long as I promised to hold onto the handrails. Becoming room free was an important milestone for me because it restored one of the freedoms I had lost. I worked at this diligently. I even cheated on occasion by practicing before I was cleared to do so. Despite my head still being heavy with the staples and my vision still being slightly blurred, I eventually was room free about 10 days after the surgery.

At the point I earned this freedom back, I was doing physical therapy twice per day and my speech and occupational therapy was down to once daily. As soon as I earned my room-free merit badge, I was getting up to use the bathroom far more often than I needed to. I continued to practice and I worked toward the day when I would be able to shower again on my own. I worked at manipulating the shower's flow settings and handling the soap all while gripping tightly on the handrails.

The therapy was having drastic positive impact on my physical condition. I was allowed to leave my room, still with the help of a walker, and visit the physical therapy gym to practice various exercises. I was no longer the new guy in the wing and I was able to move about the hospital because of my seniority. My physical therapists, Scott and Joe, were both very encouraging. When I was working with one, the other would shout motivation from across the room. They both wanted me to work hard and I wanted to be the best patient I possibly could. I had built a solid rapport with my therapists. I trusted their guidance and I looked forward to our sessions together.

Sarah continued to be direct in our meetings. Her information provided me with a baseline for my condition. The thought of how accurate Dr. Morgan was about my circumstance hours before my operation, coupled with Sarah's information, helped me to better understand my situation. Sarah and I were meeting once a day and I was as tired after her speech sessions as I was after one of my physical therapy sessions. The mental exercises Sarah administered were somewhat challenging, but did not require a high I.Q. She was aware that I was still under heavy anti-seizure medication and understood the impact it had on my ability to think as quickly as normal. Although I struggled through her puzzles, I compared them to something you might find printed along the back pages of an in-flight magazine.

Sarah recommended early on that I start writing and using notes as much as possible, for it would help spark the parts of my brain that organized information. Diligent note taking would help strengthen the mental templates in my mind, known as *schemata* in the world of psychology. Continued "memory jogging" was crucial to my mental recovery. I started making entries in my logs that soon turned into a comprehensive journal, which, collectively, soon evolved into this book. I would jot down notes every day that described, in detail, the key events, assignments, disciplines and timetables that I was exposed to daily.

Dr. Morgan was very supportive of my journal. He encouraged me to stick with it and five months after my surgery he told me I was a "poster boy" for recovery efforts. He went on to say that a large challenge for doctors in his position was convincing patients to work on physical therapy as quickly and as deliberately as possible. Dr. Morgan hoped that I would soon transform my journal into a book that others could read to find inspiration. We shared this goal. As a result of Sarah's beginning education in brain injuries, I continued to research my condition and became a lay expert in the topic. My hope is that this book can inspire *at least* one person to accelerate his or her physical therapy, speech pathology and occupational programs. If I can convince at least one person that they *can* recover, it will be worth all of my efforts.

My determination not to have a "normal" recovery program helped me stay motivated with my physical therapy. I wanted to be listed on the far right side of the bell curve and it was my intention to always do more than was expected. If Joe asked me to do 10 reps, I would make an effort to do 15 or 20. If Scott saw I was tired and recommended that I slow down or stop, I would fight to do a few more of whatever exercise I was doing at the time. My execution of the exercises was still not perfect and I stumbled on occasion. But, I was making a conscious effort to return to my pre-surgery state as soon as possible and I was doing anything to elevate my benefit.

My stay in rehab brought about a few more friendly phone conversations with Dr. Bryan and he continued to guarantee me a 100 percent recovery. I thought he might be planting the seeds for a self-fulfilling prophecy; if I expected a full recovery, then my behaviors would reflect that goal. Dr. Morgan also called to complement me on the results and reports he was receiving that outlined my progress. This was powerful validation that my approach to recovery was paying off.

Nine days after surgery, and five days into rehab, I started making the hard sale to my physical therapists that I should be going home soon. I considered myself a fairly good salesman, having attended business college while I was finishing high school. The key curriculum of business college—salesmanship—had stuck with me and paid great dividends throughout my entire life. Scott agreed to take a field trip to my house to assess the amount of risky terrain; he called it a "home audit."

On the way over I secretly wished I lived in a one-story home with gently slopping entrance ramps and patted counters. Instead, the reality was that I lived in a three-story house with a long, steep driveway and hard stone everything. Scott studied the arrangements I would be facing daily if I were to go home. We entered in through the second level and Scott examined the kitchen, family room, library and office that spanned the middle floor. Next, we traveled up the 18 stairs that led us to the bedroom suites on the third floor. One concern I had was if I would ever again be able to carry Charlie up these stairs if the sleepy guy fell asleep on one of the lower levels. While in the hospital, I often thought that in my condition I would be satisfied if I were lucky enough to simply hold his hand while we climbed the stairs.

Besides having to negotiate the flights of stairs, the bedrooms on the third level presented little problem. On the lower level, 36 stairs down from the bedrooms, Scott walked through our recreation room, guest rooms and entertainment area. After his initial assessment, Scott was deliberate in educating me about what I would be required to do to maneuver around my home. This was something I had never consciously thought about in all my years of calling this house *home*. Because Scott was ultra-sensitive about another fall, he insisted that I must not be left alone. Another fall could be detrimental now that my head was full of staples and partially formed by two metal plates.

On Sunday, November 23rd, 11 days past surgery, I was discharged from the Renown Rehabilitation Unit. But, only after all the therapists accepted my promise to honor their rules and recommendations did they allow me to climb into my getaway car with Anna. Despite the tremendous and wonderful care I was under, I was anxious to go home. Joe once said that neurological patients stay an average of 3-4 weeks, so my early release was encouraging.

While I was pleased to be going home, I was more than slightly concerned about leaving the place where skilled professionals had so closely monitored me. An assistant was always on hand if I had complications while eating, using the bathroom, doing exercises, etc. Plus, they were always near by to assist me with the problems that had developed in my urinary tract, which was another complication that arose during my hospital stay. Regrettably, I was unable to convince the supervising nurses that I could monitor my fluid retention and avoid the "dreaded tube" (urinary catheter). It was, to say the least, a very unpleasant procedure. To make matters worse, I had contracted a staph infection during the process. Although, it would prove to be another seven months until the infection completely cleared up, I was determined to get back to living in my own home.

Chapter 13

A Home Built With Milestones

A number of unforeseen challenges presented themselves soon after I was back living in my own home. I was uncomfortable having to watch Anna handle the household chores that I usually performed. I was unable to pick up any objects around the house because I could not grip them. My dexterity was greatly impaired and I felt quite awkward, even in my own home. I would slowly walk by my workshop in the garage and wonder when or *if* I would ever again be able to control my power tools. My movements were measured and planned, as I was all too aware that the slightest accident could be fatal.

One commitment I made before I left the hospital was to continue to do outpatient speech pathology and physical rehabilitation. I thought it was extremely convenient that I was able to find a quality rehab center only 10 minutes from my home. I was dedicated to work as hard as I had when I was a confined patient at the mercy of the hospital's rehabilitation staff. I was pleased to find the same level of support at my outpatient center as I had in the hospital. It was mere luck to again work with a gifted speech pathologist who took such a strong interest in my progress.

Now that I again had the freedom of living back at home, my merit badges were growing in intensity. Instead of working on Sarah's therapeutic puzzles to help regain my prioritizing and judgment skills, I was now getting close to putting them back to action in my company. Of course, the consequences of poor judgment would now cost far more than an unfavorable mark and the embarrassment of a redo.

Twenty days after surgery, I had my home office functional and semi-organized. Key executives from my company were stopping in to pay me visits. Even though many of them may have originally stopped by to express their well-wishes, we inherently resorted to business talk. I needed a benchmark to test the recovery of my mental activity. Numbers seemed to be the obvious solution because they had come natural to me since before grade school. I believed I was making steady progress, but it was impossible for me not to have private doubt about my ability to make sound business decisions.

At the time I went into surgery, our economy was 17 months into the worst downturn our country had seen since the Great Depression. Because I knew the times were dire and some major decisions needed to be made immediately, the condition of my business was constantly on my mind. I started a routine of physically going into my office and looking over reports, making phone calls and meeting with other executives. Dr. Morgan made it very clear that he only wanted me working one hour at a time and then taking time to rest. This was not always easy to do, but when someone saves your life, you tend to take their advice quite seriously. I followed his instruction closely during my first week of being home. However, on the 27th day post-surgery I was involved in a three-day complex negotiation with someone who would later turn out to be the worst of adversaries. My body was still full of hospital-administered drugs and I was taking 200 milligrams of Dilantin daily. For anyone unfamiliar with the drug, and be thankful you are, Dilantin is an anti-seizure medication with many side effects, none of them positive.

Because I was still under the spell of the heavy anti-seizure medication, Dr. Morgan had cautioned me several times against entering lengthy business negotiations without assistance. But, being an entrepreneur with a company as complex as mine, it was impossible to eliminate me from the equation and still press forward. The financial demands of my company, with the world in the fragile economic state that it was, required me to occasionally depart from Dr. Morgan's professional advice.

On December 24th, 41 days after surgery, I was released far ahead of time from my outpatient speech and occupational therapy. My gifted therapist, Nicole, requested that I keep making a conscious effort to monitor my speech and keep exercising my brain. Of course, I obliged. Back when I was released from Renown, I began struggling with the New York Times crossword puzzles and had become quite addicted. Nicole thought it would behoove me to keep working the puzzles. She also strongly encouraged me to take notes, practice organizing personal files and continue with a long list of other habitual errands, which would have all been beneficial practices sans brain surgery.

Two days after Christmas I ventured into my workshop determined to work with my power tools. I was cautious and took the necessary precautions of wearing safety glasses and protective gloves, something I had not always thought necessary pre-surgery. Handling the various drills, operating the bench saw, swinging a hammer and accurately maneuvering my automatic screwdriver dramatically boosted my confidence. Although, I must admit, I did not remember the tools making such an incredible amount of noise or moving at such sensational speeds. Nonetheless, I was excited to be using the same tools that 44 days before I was uncertain if I would ever *see* again, let alone be able to handle.

Forty-five days after surgery I decided to drive my Hummer down our driveway. Because I was still taking a strong regiment of anti-seizure medication, I had not yet been cleared to operate a vehicle—let alone a Hummer. But, I could not help myself. Even though I took enjoyment in being escorted around by the world's prettiest chauffer, Anna leads a very active life and I was eager to again be able to drive myself. I cautiously climbed in the Marine-green beast and managed the vehicle slowly and surely, lightly pressing on the brakes, carefully putting the vehicle in gear and reversing at a snail's pace. I knew I was not supposed to be driving, but I was delighted to maneuver the world's largest standard-production civilian passenger vehicle down my driveway and back. Without detection, I crawled the machine back into its spot in the garage, removed the key and delicately stepped down—all the while smiling like a teenager who just past his first driving test.

On January 2nd, I went to my scheduled electroencephalograph (more commonly referred to as an EEG) screening. The situation was puzzling. An assortment of medical professionals strategically placed 27 electronic strobes about my head. I was again back to passively lying on an apparatus at Renown Medical Center. With my eyes closed, I was able to detect what seemed to be an endless series of strobe lights. The strobes all demonstrated different patterns, each with its own meaningful purpose in evaluating my brain's responses. This was a very passive procedure; I could not influence the outcome if I tried, which meant none of my clever ways of proving I was progressing would make a difference. Thankfully, the test did not uncover anything out of the ordinary for a person at my stage of recovery.

Despite all of the positive progress I was proud to be making, my weeks were still riddled with sobering moments. At one point, 50-plus days post-surgery, Charlie ran up to me and politely asked me to knot his tie, as he was getting ready for church. After a few embarrassing attempts, I realized I had forgotten how. I have been looping ties around my neck since I was a teen, but at that point I had forgotten the seemingly mindless technique. I felt saddened and embarrassed, even though I knew Charlie was not judging me. I took refuge in my dressing room for the next 45 minutes, desperately trying to remember the simple process. The situation especially frightened me because I thought I had lost the pocket of my brain where this type of information was normally stored. However, through trial and error, I was able to reconstruct the mundane task.

I fought through similar trying instances and continued to trudge through my recovery. Early one Monday morning I convinced Anna to let me roll a large garbage receptacle down our steep driveway and onto the street. She hesitated at first, but eventually agreed. She watched me like a hawk as I slowly made my way down the pavement, which spanned approximately two blocks. I took on the smallest tasks, like taking out the trash, with confidence. Each elementary assignment boosted my morale and led the way to more sophisticated ones.

On January 7th I completed my formal physical therapy. Thankfully, my progress had exceeded the clinic's expectations and they released me early—again, only if I promised to continue with their prescribed activities.

Two days after completing outpatient physical therapy, Dr. Morgan made the decision to reduce my anti-seizure regiment to half of the previous amount. Almost immediately after the reduction, I detected a notable difference in regards to my responsiveness. My legs seemed steadier, my arms were reacting quicker and my hand activity was more precise. All of these active functions were welcomed, but I was concerned that the reduction in medication could attract another seizure. I had to put my faith in Dr. Morgan, as I had through this entire ordeal. To my delight, I was also authorized to drive again. I would miss having my lovely wife chauffer me around, but I was very pleased to once again have the freedoms that came with being able to drive myself.

Whether he realized it or not, Charlie had been an incredible motivator for my recovery. While still in the ICU I had thought about how badly I still wanted to be capable of carrying Charlie up the stairs to his bed after he fell asleep. Soon after I moved back home I would convince Charlie that he was helping *me* up the stairs when we would travel them to his bedroom together, hand-in-hand. It was greatly satisfying, but I was not yet confident that I could lug him up the flight if he had fallen asleep while watching TV with me downstairs.

I was eager to get back to the activities we had enjoyed together before my operation. We always liked being outside on sunny days and 57 days post-op I was able to again take my son to a nearby park. We had a wonderful time peddling about on our tandem bicycle (pictured later in the photo section of this book). I was in front and Charlie, my co-pilot, helped us along in the back. With cautious ease, we circled the park's quarter-mile track four times. I had the feeling that Charlie was pleased that his father was again able to participate in normal, fun activities. Later in the afternoon, we were both excited to shoot hoops and continue enjoying our time together on a particularly sunny winter day. I brought a ladder along to level the playing field for Charlie. Perched on the ladder, Charlie would sling the ball at the basket a few yards away and I would collect the rebound to either take a shot or hand it back. With the height disadvantage eliminated, we made about the same number of baskets and shot a pretty even game.

January 13th marked the 60th day since my surgery. I was delighted this day because I finally finished for my sister Pat the birdhouse that had ailed me while lying immobile on the hospital bed. The hurricane-proof bird mansion was on the way to its new home and I was very pleased to finish one of the projects that had been on my mind since the surgery. I remember back to my days in the ICU when I would think about the birdhouse and did not know if I would ever be able to handle the craftsmanship it required. I was very grateful to finish the birdhouse because it meant I had regained some of the skills that I valued so dearly.

January 19th, 66 days post-surgery, brought about a number of memorable milestones. My anti-seizure medication was discontinued and I felt comfortable driving both day and night. My company was moving forward through the difficult economic times and I felt like my business activity was making progress with each week. Feeling confident with my abilities, I reassumed the responsibilities of the CEO and CFO positions. Before reassuming the roles, I had placed a dramatic expense-reduction policy into effect. Up to the point of writing this book, the initiative has amounted to over $13 million, which is a huge cut in a company the size of mine.

The same day I stepped back into the positions, I was also able, for the first time, to carry Charlie up two flights of stairs after he fell asleep. I was very careful to take one step at a time with the sleepy guy in my arms, his head cradled between my neck and shoulder. Carrying Charlie to bed marked another feat I was concerned with while in the ICU and it was a symbolic accomplishment to have the strength to do so. At the top of the stairs Charlie whispered, "You are really strong." I tucked this merit badge in my back pocket, knowing I would hold onto its personal meaning for the rest of my life.

Chapter 14

Taking Chances

My great nephew Erik is an exceptional teenage hockey player. He is very connected with the sport and I had promised his grandfather I would acquire and send to him a framed and signed Wayne Gretzky jersey. Gretzky's number 99 is the only number to ever be retired across an entire sport. The Great One's impact on hockey was legendary. I remembered a quote I valued from Gretzky in which he said, "You miss 100 percent of the shots you never take." I was happy to send the jersey to Erik and hoped it would encourage him to take chances, both on the ice and off. Erik's grandfather, my only brother, is a retired Marine Lt Col and easily ranks at the top of my all-time hero list. I have a tremendous deal of respect and admiration for him and I was honored to send a meaningful token to his grandson.

On January 28th I took a trip to the Renown Rehabilitation Unit to visit my three therapist heroes: Joe, Scott and Sarah. We had a warm, endearing conversation in which they told me collectively that they had believed if anyone had the discipline to make a full recovery, it was me. Their comments showed their support for me and their sincerity was clear when they each individually reiterated the same message to me later. I was flattered when Sarah said I looked "full of life" and Joe said it was as if "the surgery had never happened."

I wore my leather bomber jacket and they remembered how when I was in the hospital I had worn an assortment of Marine Corps hats and T-shirts. I told them I did so because I believed they served as reminders of the discipline and focus I learned in the Corps. The reminders allowed me to apply these traits to my early recovery.

On February 20th I had a sit-down meeting with Dr. Morgan. At this point he felt I had recovered enough to delve into the seriousness of my situation. Dr. Morgan was a very diplomatic and tactful surgeon. His readiness to discuss my ordeal in detail showed me he was comfortable with my present condition. The CAT scans were showing no issues of concern after the surgery. He encouraged me to continue recording my log and again strongly suggested that I eventually turn my journals into a book.

Every day since I had been released from the hospital I had worked at returning to normalcy. I made countless short-term goals and aimed to achieve them one at a time. I was grateful for all the mobility that I had regained and I was pleased to be spending time with my lovely family. Despite my progress, I still had the uncomfortable feeling of not being completely back to what I considered normal. Although I tried to practice patience, my shortcomings still bothered me. For instance, Anna had filmed some family footage around Christmas. She videotaped Charlie opening presents on Christmas Day, which was 42 days post-surgery. I did not watch the footage until months after the occasion, but when I did I was saddened by my condition in the video. At the time I felt like I was making a sizeable effort to return to normal, but looking back I saw I was a long way from it. My eyes looked droopy, my movements appeared sluggish and all together I looked like someone that needed help with the simplest tasks. When I first saw the family footage, I wanted to blame the seizure medication for my slothful look. But, I had to understand that the person on the video was in normal condition for someone who had undergone an invasive brain surgery one-and-one-half months earlier.

Every day I tried to progress, even though it was trying on my patience. In yet another effort to regain a part of my life that I had enjoyed prior to the surgery, I decided to drive to Mount Rose Ski Resort on a snowy Sunday morning. I packed my snow-ski equipment into the Hummer and drove by myself to the mountain. When I arrived, I pulled into a handicapped parking spot and stepped into the thin mountain air—all 19 degrees of it. I was nervous because I knew I was pushing my boundaries, even though it had been 93 days since my surgery. In the parking lot I wrestled with my ski boots, which teamed with the cold wind to put up quite the battle. The clunky plastic ski boots had a series of stubborn snaps that, one by one, I managed to force into place. My new specialized helmet was heavier than a normal helmet, but I still feared bumping my head on the ground, or a tree, or another skier. The whole process of snapping into my gear and hauling my skis to the ski area was challenging and tiring. Along the hike, I questioned my wisdom several times for what I was about to do.

I stepped into my skis and attempted to get used to the feeling. I traversed up the hill a ways to try my luck heading back down a slow run in the beginners' area (I preferred to think of it as a *beginners' area* rather than a *bunny slope*). I stayed in this area for two hours and soon I felt comfortable with the idea of heading to one of the ski lifts. However, since I was alone and would soon be feeling the fatigue, I decided to pass on the idea. The idea of an accident was too much. I was proud with my efforts and was pleased to live to ski another day. This benchmark day was validating for my approach to normalcy.

February 28th, 2009 was Charlie's sixth birthday. Our house was filled with excitement and I was pleased to share the day with Charlie trying out the new remote-controlled racetrack I had bought for him. The race set came with pages upon pages of instructions for its assembly. I retreated alone to a room to work on piecing it together; I figured revealing the final project to Charlie would be more exciting than handing him a box filled with various plastic parts, screws and cellophane-wrapped race cars. I knew assembling the track would not be too challenging after all my experience working with wood and power tools. As I clicked and screwed the plastic pieces together, I remember what a great day it was in physical therapy when they incorporated the use of screws and bolts into my regiment. I was always pleased when they introduced something that related to my *real* life outside of the hospital. After completing the racetrack, Charlie and I raced matchbox-sized cars through the turns and tunnels for the better part of his birthday afternoon.

Chapter 15

Picking Up The Pace

My running routine was one thing I had not revisited enough post-surgery to be satisfied. However, I was slowly getting back to running on my treadmill. On March 7th I was able to run five-and-one-half miles, which was the most I had completed since before my operation. I was pleased with this feat even though it was minor when compared to the lengths of runs I was used to. I often found it challenging to avoid comparing my capacity post-operation to my capacity pre-operation. Remembering to keep progressing was crucial, and still is. With the help of my treadmill, I made an effort to continue working on improving my running; I desperately wanted it to again be part of my regular exercise routine.

My responsibilities within my company continued to pick up and with Dr. Morgan's blessing I was traveling by air for a number of required business ventures. I also was fortunate to fly with Charlie across the country during a trip to see my mother. We flew from Reno to Atlanta and then drove the two hours to Oxford, Alabama. Charlie makes an excellent traveling buddy; he was content on the flight and patient on the drive.

The day after stopping in Oxford we set off toward our home in Pensacola, Florida where Anna was already waiting for us. The drive took five hours and Charlie and I enjoyed nice conversations in between the times he could not help but succumb to the lure of short road-trip naps. When he would awaken, we would pick up right where we left off, with me answering his seemingly endless series of questions, which I loved.

The seven total hours of driving required an amount of alertness I had not particularly paid attention to in the past. Thankfully, the traffic problems were fairly mild and my copilot and I traveled with relative ease. When we crossed the Florida border we began to smell the thick salty air and I had the most pleasant feeling of being back in the area where I grew up. I was eager to get to my home in Pensacola, which 120 days prior I did not know if I would ever visit again. Anna had reached our home a few days earlier to stock the house with provisions and she was delighted to see the two of us pull into the driveway.

The next day brought about a soft warm March rain that lasted through the evening. To the surprise of some of my neighbors, I decided to take a short run in the light rain. I was thrilled to run in the warm air and grateful to have the mobility to quickly place one foot after the other to the pavement. On the three-mile run I did not encounter any obstacles, but along the last four months, I knew I had overcome many. I was lucky to be alive, to be running in the rain, to be traveling and to be again spending time with those I loved. As I thought about how fortunate I was, the run quickly became the most satisfying trek in my entire running career.

After our trip to Florida, we made it back to Reno and reassumed our daily activities. Charlie and I again went to shoot hoops and I focused on taking shots with my left hand, knowing that my brain problem had affected my left side more significantly. After four months of recovering I was able to recognize a notable difference in my left hand dexterity. My therapy had targeted both, but it took longer for the function in my left side to catch up to that of my right.

By the first quarter of business, on March 30th, 2009, I was delighted that my company's operating profits were up 17 percent, which was a counter trend to most businesses at the time.

I was also working on getting my running routine back to a consistent trend when my treadmill, which had been faithful for more than 20 years, seized up and died. After becoming certain the old beast was shot, I quickly went out to buy a new one. The sports store I went to had the treadmill I wanted, but they charged a $125 assembly fee. I was quickly turned off by the idea of paying someone to put it together. Plus, in my Hummer, I could not transport a fully assembled treadmill back home. So, I decided to purchase the new treadmill unassembled and challenge myself to piece together the complex machine. I wanted to show the old treadmill respect by taking it apart piece by piece myself, and I could send it out with the weekly trash if it was completely disassembled. After several hours working with my wrenches, screwdrivers, hammers and other hand tools, my hand dexterity was validated. I disassembled my veteran 20-year-old treadmill and gave it a customary trash-bin burial. Two days later I had my new treadmill assembled and running smoothly; I continue to use it to this day.

On May 5th, I had a regular visit with Dr. Bryan. I checked in at 147 pounds, up from 138 in the hospital. I felt good about recovery and I was inspired to take on more physical activity, which improved my health. My blood pressure was 120 over 80 and my cholesterol was 131. Dr. Bryan joked with me that if all of his patients were in my condition, he would be out of a job. Dr. Bryan was good-natured and he always boosted my morale. I always took his advice seriously and followed it as closely as I could.

Six months after my operation, Anna and I took Charlie to El Capitan Resort and Casino in Hawthorne, Nevada. An armed forces parade was scheduled to take place on Saturday, May 16th. Charlie was asked to ride on a float and throw out candy to spectators. I was on the reviewing stand when Charlie's float passed and I was very proud of how considerate Charlie was. Occasionally, Charlie would spot a veteran in a wheelchair and he was very deliberate to jump down and run over to place a piece of candy in the veteran's hand. Having watched my recovery very closely, Charlie knew it would be difficult for injured vets to catch candy on the fly. He exhausted himself making sure every disabled person along the float trail had candy. Many times the vets would salute to

Charlie and, having practiced his right-hand address for months, he would snap a satisfying salute right back to them.

Ten days later, on Memorial Day, I proudly put on my Marine Corps dress blues for Charlie (pictured in the photo section). It took little effort but it was another gratifying gesture I had been aching to do since lying helpless in the ICU. Not to make you old vets feel jealous, but my dress blue uniform still fit me well. It felt good to put them on for Charlie, but it also felt good for me. The Marines will always be important to me. The Corps deepened my discipline and indisputably helped save my life many times. No matter what happens, I will always be a Marine.

Chapter 16

Business as Unusual

Thinking back to the summer of 2008, things were happening to me that had me silently concerned about my failing health. My condition was yet to be accurately diagnosed as my strength began to gradually fade away. To complicate matters further, my company's major bank failed; this was July 25th, 2008, only four months prior to my being rushed into emergency brain surgery. The failed bank was taken over by the Federal Deposit Insurance Corporation (FDIC). The bank, which had been thrown into limbo, was holding a loan that was intrinsically important to my company. Since I was sole shareholder of the company, the matter imprisoned a great deal of my attention.

Up until the time I was admitted to the hospital, and immediately into surgery, on November 13th, 2008, I had presented a steady stream of plans to the FDIC to completely retire the loan. The loan was secured by six operating casinos, which in fact were the largest part of my 10-casino enterprise. I wanted to protect those assets because they represented a key component of my estate. The bankers at the former bank knew this. Once my loan was thrown in with hundreds of other business' loans and swallowed by the FDIC and delegated contractors, I made sure the FDIC understood the situation.

The FDIC has volumes of guidelines and regulations to conduct an orderly and fair disposition and resolution of loans. I was under the assumption that my loan would be fairly handled according to the FDIC's strict guidelines. Little did I know that unethical individuals and rogue bankers were singling out my loan. They unlawfully manipulated the FDIC's established policies and rushed my loan through a clandestine backroom maze of FDIC violations, all the while denying and ignoring my rights. All of this scampering was to achieve the end result of scoring my company's $66 million-plus pool of assets. They took the pool of assets, which held a future discounted value of over $100 million, from my company and sold it to their friends for a net price of $5.8 million. In the end, these people's dirty hands greased their own pockets with millions of illegal dollars.

During the heart of their effort, they did have and added advantage: I was fighting for my life and uncertain future, if I had any future at all. I am positive the rumors of my dying gave them added confidence. With my life being compromised by a traumatic head injury, their scheme could be pulled off and this group would be handsomely enriched at the expense of the FDIC and my family. It appeared so easy for them, dealing with what looked to be a dying and/or permanently impaired entrepreneur. The simplest way to describe my adversaries in their effort to steal my properties is to say they behaved as schoolyard bullies.

> *"You and your company have been victimized with the worst abuse, illegal manipulation and criminal conduct that I have seen in my over 30 years of practice."*
> —Attorney (who will go unnamed), Washington, D.C.

As these crooks' attempt to rob me was becoming very clear, I was under my neurosurgeon's instructions that permitted me to work only an hour at a time and rest often. He highly discouraged me from making any major financial decisions. While his instructions inhibited my ability to perform and protect my business, they were understandable. Each day, remember, I was taking 100 mgs of the anti-seizure drug Dilantin, which comes with a pleasant list of common side effects including slurred speech, confusion and sporadic eye movements. On December 11th, only a few days released from the hospital, my adversaries demanded a meeting, supposedly to complete a *friendly* deal. However, as I later discovered, the meeting was a ruse to conceal their unlawful due diligence and assist them in acquiring a loan to make their unlawful purchase of my loan.

My skull was still unsightly red with 39 metal scalp staples holding my incision closed. As much as possible, I tried to conceal my weakened condition.

I was still unsteady on my feet as I relearned to walk. I would take frequent restroom breaks and grab pieces of candy for energy. I was sucking it up, constantly reminding myself that I am a Marine. They, on the other hand, were unrelenting. The meeting lasted three days. I told no one about the meeting, most assuredly my surgeon; I knew if he found out he would send me back to hospital. I had to go to bed for two full days after they left. As I slept, they went to Las Vegas to meet with the rogue bankers and continue the scheme.

I am not going to let the crap you're going through now define your distinguished career."
-Anna Maria Holder, Wife

On February 4th, 2009, I got a call from the group that claimed they purchased my loan. However, they could not show me any written proof of the purchase. They told me they wanted to foreclose on me in five days. Both the group and the rogue bankers claimed to be surprised after getting a $2.5 million discount (a.k.a. gift from the FDIC) on a loan they also had in the same loan portfolio of the failed bank. This occurred December 15th, 2008, the same day the pool of loans, which I understood my loan was in, was scheduled to be sold. My loan had been mysteriously pulled from the sale and handled in secret, following the same pattern of criminal conduct that had advanced the scam to this point. This was all done in violation of federal laws and long standing FDIC operating procedures and guidelines. The setup for a special-treatment handling of my loan and the illegal sale thereafter greatly enriched the purchasers and their associates by millions of dollars. The FDIC and, more importantly, my family were the ones footing the bill.

"A 12-inch stack of legal documents as protection will not protect you from crooks. A single page of the same is all one needs from an honest person."
-Jim Moore, Seasoned Professional Banker

No knowledgeable person I know feels this situation was anything but an illegally stacked deck and circumnavigation of established laws, which all ended in criminal enrichment. Normally, I would welcome the challenges presented by a shaky economy and competitive opponents. However, dealing with dishonest and unethical adversaries significantly tilts the playing field in their favor and taints business operations. I am trying to protect the family assets I have earned throughout a lifetime of hard honest work and it is extremely frustrating when those attempting to take them behave illegally. I never have asked for anything to be given to me, nor have I asked for a given quarter because of brain-surgery impairment. I know I disappointed the "bullies," their attorneys and their associates by not dying.

"My brain is my capital."
-Ernest Hemingway

The investigation into the illegal scheme, which turned my life upside down, has uncovered a mountain of evidence supporting wrongdoings and unlawful criminal acts. On December 20th, 2010 my company filed a federal lawsuit in Reno for over $60 million in monetary damages. We will also seek punitive and other damages. Like my physical recovery from brain surgery, the federal lawsuit is still a work in progress.

Chapter 17

The Slow Process

by Anna Holder

———•———

One month before Harold's emergency operation, I was working in our home office when I was startled by a large thump. I hurried toward the garage where Harold and Charlie were spending time together. Harold was spread on the floor at the foot of the stairs. He had evidently come back into the house and tried to go upstairs; he did not make it. I rolled him over on his back. He was barely lucid. His breathing was OK, but he was definitely out of it. Despite his condition, he still asked about Charlie; Harold was concerned that Charlie would walk in and find him in his fragile state.

Immediately, I called 9-1-1. When the ambulance got to the house the paramedics took Harold to the Renown Medical branch closest to our home. After running a number of tests the doctors attributed the fall to bacterial pneumonia, which is known to cause sporadic drops in blood pressure and would explain Harold's dizziness just before he fell. The doctor prescribed intravenous antibiotics and insisted that Harold stay at the hospital overnight for monitoring. Charlie and I brought him some of his toiletries, newspapers and snacks. I noticed that Harold was uncharacteristically weak. The doctors released him the next day and Harold agreed to take it easy around the house while he recovered from the "pneumonia."

After returning home, Harold never seemed to totally recover. I attributed his constant fatigue to the stress of his work. Harold was facing some of the most difficult challenges of his business career. When coupled with the disloyalty from some of his colleagues, dishonesty and harassment from others, I thought his tiredness was completely due to work. It never occurred to me that something more serious was going on.

Weeks later, on November the 13th, I remember Harold waking up in the middle of the night, stumbling and struggling to get back into bed. The entire left side of his body seemed limp, but because he was alert and coherent, he convinced me that he was fine. Regardless, I watched him throughout the rest of the night. He was breathing fine and appeared to be sleeping comfortably. When he awoke again he was feeling better. However, I knew something was off; I just could not put my finger on it.

I waited until 7 a.m. and right on the dot I called Dr. Richard Bryan. He listened to me explain what I saw going on with Harold and he responded in a more serious tone. He said it sounded neurological and told me that he would call Renown and let the doctors know we were coming and which tests needed to be performed. Dr. Bryan could not see Harold because he was on his way to his clinic in

Bishop, California. Plus, by the sound of Dr. Bryan's assumptions, it was not anything a cardiologist could diagnose anyhow.

Harold insisted on going about his morning routine. He showered, had his coffee and went about his day as if everything was normal. I dropped Charlie off at school and when I returned I convinced Harold to leave for Renown Urgent Care, even though he seemed to be lacking urgency. It was about 9 a.m. when Harold checked in and waited to undergo the tests Dr. Bryan had recommended. After lunch Harold prepared for a CAT scan. Around 2:30 we did not have any results so I left momentarily to go pick up Charlie.

On my way to Charlie's school I received a phone call from the doctor who was attending to Harold. She said they were sending him to the main hospital because they had found something serious. Because of the urgent tone in her voice, I decided to leave Charlie at school instead of bringing him to the hospital.

On my way downtown to Renown Medical Center I got a call from Bryce Munson, M.D., a friend of ours who is a doctor at Renown Urgent Care. She asked me where Charlie was. When I told her I left him at school she told me to quickly get to the hospital and she would send her husband to pick up Charlie. Without giving specifics, she reiterated the seriousness of the situation when I inquired why. She was extremely concerned about Charlie being able to see his father before he underwent surgery. When Bryce made it very clear that Charlie *needed* to see his father before surgery, I knew the situation was deeply serious.

When I got to the hospital, Harold was in a room with Dr. Jay Morgan, who was explaining exactly what was going on and what needed to be done immediately. He pulled me outside to tell me that anything I had to say to my husband I should say now, and quickly. Dr. Morgan informed me that he would not know what he could do until he physically got inside Harold's head. He said that postponing surgery was an option but he strongly suggested against it because, if not operated on, Harold could be dead by the next day.

I went back into the room with Harold and we quickly agreed that surgery was the right option. When Charlie arrived, we explained the best we could that the doctors needed to operate on his father's brain. Charlie briefly sat with Harold before leaving to spend the rest of the evening at a friend's house. He did not quite understand the severity of the moment but at least he got to see his father and hug him before Harold was taken away for surgery.

Harold started to cry gently and told me he was sorry and that he did not want to leave me this way. I told him that he was a good man, a good father and a good husband. I tried to reassure him that Charlie and I would be fine and that he needed to concentrate on surgery. I reiterated that everything was going to be fine and I would see him after the surgery.

It is rather numbing to be told that your husband is in serious condition and probably will not survive surgery. My conversation with Harold was most difficult because it is one you never anticipate having with your spouse. At 5:30 p.m. Harold was wheeled back for surgery.

Two hours later I left to pick up Charlie. We picked up something to eat and briefly stopped by our home to walk the dog and try to restore a bit of normalcy. When we returned to the hospital, Charlie and I sat in the waiting room awaiting word from Dr. Morgan. Charlie quickly fell asleep on one of the couches. I looked at him while he slept and wondered what I was going to tell the little guy if Dr. Morgan came out with the worst possible news. I was running every scenario through my mind when Dr. Morgan came into the waiting room about 9:30 p.m. He told me that the pressure from the fluid had been alleviated and Harold's brain reacted in every way he had hoped for during the surgery. I was grateful for the uplifting news. We were not allowed to see Harold so I woke Charlie, shared the information with him and we went home with plans of returning the next day.

By morning, Harold had been moved to the Intensive Care Unit, which is a very sobering place because most patients are comatose. Harold's head was wrapped in bandages and an assortment of tubes sprung from underneath the wrapping. He appeared to be in a very fragile state. Charlie soaked in the circumstance the best he could and for the most part he seemed to be comfortable with it. He was chatty with his father despite the fright that you would expect drainage tubes and various machines would bring to a small child.

Harold was coherent, but the combination of the intrusive brain surgery, the morphine and the lingering anesthesia made it impossible for him to make controlled movements. He could muster the energy to speak in brief sentences. "I'm an invalid," he snapped at one point when his frustration got the best of him.

As he was unable to feed himself, I fed him and his appetite seemed good. Harold was in and out of consciousness, but each time he awoke Charlie and I were there beside him, even after visiting hours were officially over.

The next day Harold did something that proved to me his mental state was going to be fine. When the head nurse entered the room, I introduced myself. However, according to Harold, I had made a mispronunciation. I argued that I was correct and he argued back. When we asked for the nurse's opinion, she said that, in fact, Harold was correct. This was the first time I can ever remember being happy that my husband had argued with me. It was at that point when I realized he had not lost his mental ability in the surgery. I was amazed that within 48 hours of serious brain surgery, Harold regained the mental capacity to be correcting my grammar.

Physically, Harold was completely helpless. He could not feed himself or even raise a cup to his lips to drink. He could not press the button to summon the nurse and, worst of all, he could not push the button to release morphine from his drip. I knew he was in severe pain and while he had some pain meds being delivered via the IV, the head nurse made it very clear that he would *need* his morphine. The other meds were too mild to reduce his pain, so I watched the clock and periodically pushed his morphine button for him.

Later in the day the nurses removed his head wrapping to reveal a lengthy incision held together by massive staples. These staples were serious. They were the kind you would use if you had to staple a novel together. I held a mirror for Harold so he could get a visual of what he was feeling on the top of his head; it was not a pretty sight. His wounds were rather grotesque but at the same time quite amazing in the name of modern medical practices.

By day three Harold wanted to try things. He wanted to try and walk to the bathroom on his own. He wanted to try his own hand exercises to impress the nurses next time they checked the ability of his hands. What little he could do, he was doing. He was frustrated with the slow progression, but I kept reminding him that the large dose of drugs in his system was still wearing off. At one point Harold wanted to use the bathroom, a real bathroom. The catheter and bedpans were humbling and humiliating to him. I waited outside while a nurse brought a walker into the room. Two nurses attempted to help Harold off the bed and into the walker, but they were not strong enough to lift him themselves. When they requested more help, a male nurse arrived and the three of them assisted Harold to the walker. He tried so hard and got about 12 feet from his room before draining his energy. He could see the bathroom just a short distance away, but he simply could not go any farther. As the nurses turned him around to head back to his bed, I could see the disappointment on his face.

Five days after his operation, Harold got a boost of confidence when the doctors cleared him to be relocated to the rehabilitation center. Although his mobility was limited, he was moving forward in his progress. I was happy for him because I knew this was a big step toward his recovery. Harold is a doer and he was anxious to start *doing* anything.

Upon arrival Harold was insistent in starting an exercise regiment straight away. His first few days in rehab were trying and I could tell they were tiring him out. After all, he had spent the last five days bedridden and required full assistance. Now he was trying to do activities on his own without that assistance. I remember visiting him one day in rehab when he was doing his occupational therapy. I will never forget an exercise in which Harold was requested to screw and unscrew a number of hand bolts located directly above where he stood. The bolts and screws were all different shapes and sizes and they could only go into their matching holes. Bolt after bolt, Harold selected them from the table and screwed them in overhead without ever being rejected by a misshaped hole. Harold's precision meant so much to me because it reminded me of the kind of activities he excelled at before his surgery.

His mental function was nearly back to normal and now his physical condition was improving exponentially. Soon Harold was allowed to leave his room to do some of the exercises without supervision, which he seemed to be very proud of. Accompanied by his physical therapist, we took a few walks around the perimeter of the facility after I would bring him lunch. He was walking with better balance, especially when taking into account the uneven ground that ran parallel with the sidewalk.

His progress with his physical rehabilitation had the doctors considering his release. First, of course, they had to visit our home and inspect it for safety precautions, which they went over with me extensively. Thankfully, Harold was allowed to come home and be with his family before the Thanksgiving holiday. Needless to say, we had a *lot* to be thankful for.

Like each of his new environments, Harold took a couple of days to get comfortable. I remember how careful he was around the house. He saw everything as a process with certain, specific steps that had to be completed before he could move to the next. When he brushed his teeth he would carefully take hold of the toothpaste, then he would place his toothbrush by the sink. He would deliberately unscrew the toothpaste cap and place it on the counter, and so on. The processes that seemed to be one fluid step pre-surgery became a series of 15-to-20 challenging steps for him. He was very precise in everything that he did. It was as if he was carefully reprogramming himself to correctly complete the everyday tasks the rest of us take for granted. Harold was quietly re-identifying what kind of man he would be; what kind of husband; what kind of father.

Because Harold was not allowed to drive while taking the anti-seizure medication, I happily drove him to his outpatient physical therapy for every appointment. At this point his therapy was mostly organization-oriented. The therapists would ask Harold to complete exercises that helped him collect information, organize it and make sense of it. He would get angry if he missed something, which showed how seriously he was taking his continued therapy. One of his exercises put him in a situation where his children were each committed to different daily activities. Harold had to look at a weekly schedule and figure out how to allot enough time to get each child to his or her destination without any interference. I found the exercise humorous because the therapist was basically asking Harold to be me.

During the weeks following his surgery, I watched Harold go through three distinct phases: Anger, frustration and acceptance. These phases overlapped. There were still bouts of frustration and anger well after he had clearly accepted his situation once he was undergoing rehabilitation. As he began to better understand his physical capabilities, he was able to take things slower and embrace his patience.

Harold knew he was making progress, but he was eager to be back to full health. Everything was ritualistic and took him three times longer than it had pre-surgery. However, his memory was razor sharp and his mental function was nearly 100 percent. This was both a blessing and a curse because as soon as he realized his mental capacity was up to speed he started aching to get back in the office.

Even though I was fearful of leaving Harold alone, he proved to be fine. His actions showed that he did not need to be mothered; rather he just needed his family's support. Harold has never been one to ask for help, so it was difficult to determine when to intervene and when to let him struggle with the circumstance alone. However, over the years Harold has proved to me that he is terrific about knowing what his limits are. I remember when we were dating and he would take me up flying. If the weather was not perfect, if the wind was marginal, he would make the judgment call not to go. I knew that Harold, although frustrated to the point of being impatient, would not break his limits before he felt confident.

With time my husband approached closer and closer to the man he was pre-surgery. He has always been extremely disciplined with his diet and physical health. I believe his life habits earned him the opportunity to go through such a serious surgery and make such a substantial recovery.

Every once in a while, when he is relaxed, his fingers will twitch, which reminds us of the surgery he underwent. Our family will never forget how blessed we are to have Harold back. We verbalize how grateful we are every morning before breakfast. The months surrounding the surgery were emotionally trying, but the situation was very real and we were forced to deal with it the best we could. Without his courage and relentless motivation, our family would not be as strong as it is today.

Chapter 18

Observations From The Editor

By Bill M. West

In June of 2009 I received my first phone call from Harold Holder. He spoke clearly and had a deep voice that was smothered in a southern drawl that made it appear he was talking slower than he actually was. He had requested my contact information from a mutual friend whose book I had helped to compile. Hal was quick to the point and I feverishly scribbled in my notebook. Looking back to that notebook, my notes read:

> *Brain surgery, no, bacterial pnemonia (sic), no, brain surgery. 155 IQ, like to come out the same. Working title: Please Leave the Lights On. Successful operation. Cover story in a number of magazines.*
>
> *Background in Military. Always thinking and remembering. Get brain-damaged people moving again.*

During that first phone conversation he had briefly mentioned such an array of key points from his life that I figured he was either 200 years old or full of shit. I remember wondering, "Is this guy pulling my leg?" According to his claim, seven months prior he had survived a brain injury that has higher than a 50% mortality rate. In that time he had returned to speaking, walking, running, bicycling, snow skiing, playing basketball, driving Hummers, wielding power tools, operating a business and traveling cross country. *Sure.*

The month before our conversation he had been traveling for business and met the head of the cardiovascular center at Boston University on his returning flight. This doctor had been impressed with Hal's story and encouraged him to write a book, something Hal had already started. Now, he was calling me to help him organize it. I was intrigued.

For our first face-to-face meeting, Hal invited me to his office on the third floor of the Silver Club Casino. Along the walls were a variety of plaques, pictures and awards commemorating Hal on some of his most notable achievements. One-by-one the awards solidified a number of the claims he had made over the phone. It took me about six seconds to realize Hal was extremely accomplished.

As Hal began telling me his story in more detail than was possible on the phone, I detected a disconnect between the person he was talking about and the person who was talking. Though he had the scar on his closely-shaven head to prove the surgery, I did not believe that the ramifications of such a complicated brain surgery could be so concealed. He spoke clearly, walked briskly and stayed on task.

We talked about the project and the progress he had made in building the book from his collection of journal entries he had made since his surgery. I was compelled by his story and interested in learning more. We planned to schedule a meeting at his home; Hal was excited to show me his library.

Because we share the same birthday, Hal and I are exactly 52 years apart. Our reading interests only differ slightly, and we both share a passion for the written word. He collected first edition prints, many of them signed. Names such as Hemingway, Orwell, Mitchell and Fitzgerald were scribbled across the inner covers of the literary classics that lined Hal's shelves. He fingered through first editions and told me stories about how he had tracked down the works of some of his most cherished authors. His books were neatly organized and created a mosaic of visual information. We took seats across from each other at a large table in the center of his library—the creative genius of the greatest authors of the past century looking over us.

From that meeting forward, Hal and I worked at building his journal logs into this book. However, just over a month into the process, Hal started becoming less and less available because of mounting concerns with the stability of The Holder Group. I shared his interest in publishing this book as soon as possible, as I believe it is an incredible story of recovery. But, I understood his business was being threatened and his time and focus were occupied.

About every two months Hal would send me a brief email:

Bill:

*I will call you for next week,
because of the court filings,
my scheduling is out of my
control.*

*Thanks for understanding,
Hal*

Another two months would pass:

Dear Bill:

*We must move this project along.
I will call you.
Thanks for understanding, I am
living in a financial purgatory as
well as many others. It is more
than demanding and time consuming.*

*Sincerely,
Hal*

Through the challenging times, we made slow progress, with bursts of production coming sporadically when circumstances allowed us to meet. There were times when he was forced to abandon our meetings minutes before the scheduled times and I could tell the perpetual pull of the financial and legal matters were weighing on him. However, he never appeared to let them consume him during our meetings. We both knew this project had potential and worked together to complete it, all the while knowing the troubling situation that Hal was in could not keep his story from being told.

During my first visit to the Holder home, Hal gave me a copy of his first book, 1975's *Don't Shoot, I'm Only a Trainee*, first edition. It was signed to me and dated. Over the next few days I read through *Don't Shoot*, always seeing Hal's best wishes on the inside cover. As I helped Hal collect facts, rifle through notes and organize this book, I always kept the copy of *Don't Shoot* near the computer where I write. It acted as continuous motivation, always reminding me that one day soon Hal would invite me over to his home and hand me a signed copy of *Please Leave the Lights On*.

Hal's story is enduring and it has been an honor to work with him on this book. How he was able to dedicate time to its completion amidst the financial thunderstorm he was going through is beyond me. Once the dust clears I hope he can find the time to promote this book and get it into the hands of those who can find motivation from its contents. Its message resonates with those either facing a difficult recovery themselves or helping a loved one to press forward through one.

ACCOMPANYING PHOTOGRAPHS

I'm always smiling when in the cockpit as pilot in command. Pictured here in an SN-J Warbird.

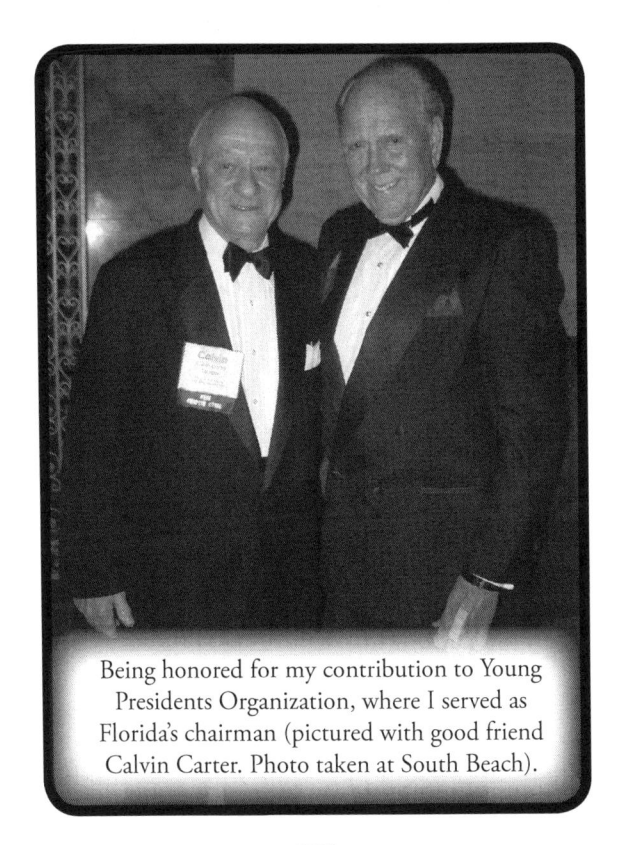

Being honored for my contribution to Young Presidents Organization, where I served as Florida's chairman (pictured with good friend Calvin Carter. Photo taken at South Beach).

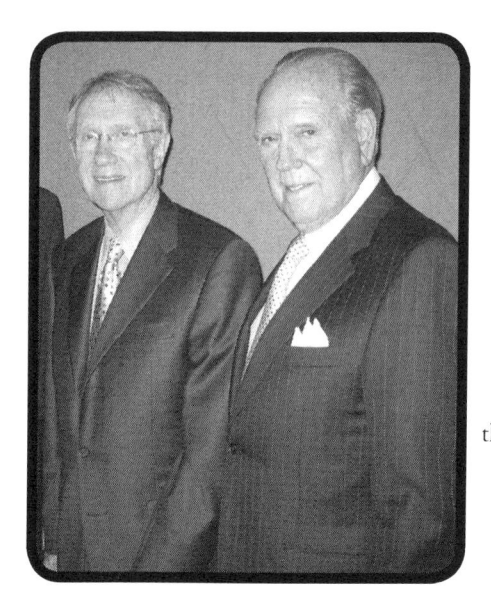

Pictured here with Senator Harry Reid, who was very supportive of me during my recovery. The senator was also helpful in bringing to the attention of government agencies the mistreatment of me and my company.

Pulling my son Charlie in his sled after a Reno snowstorm. This is the same driveway I slipped and bounced my head off of during an icy January dawn in 2004, which could have been the start of my developing hematoma.

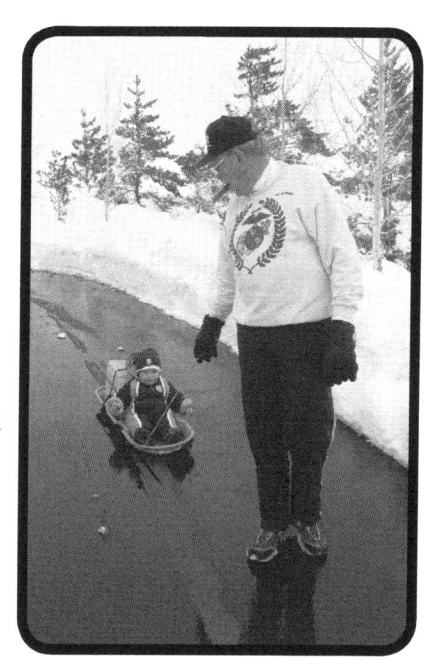

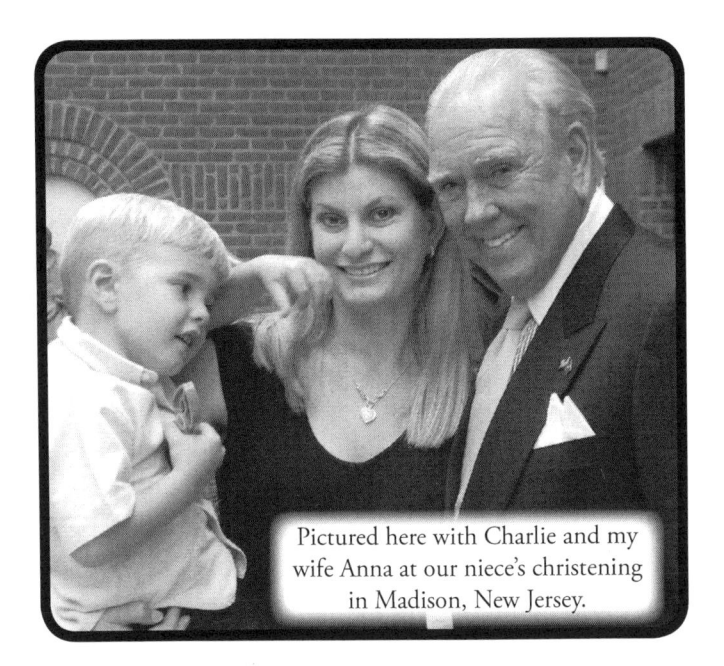

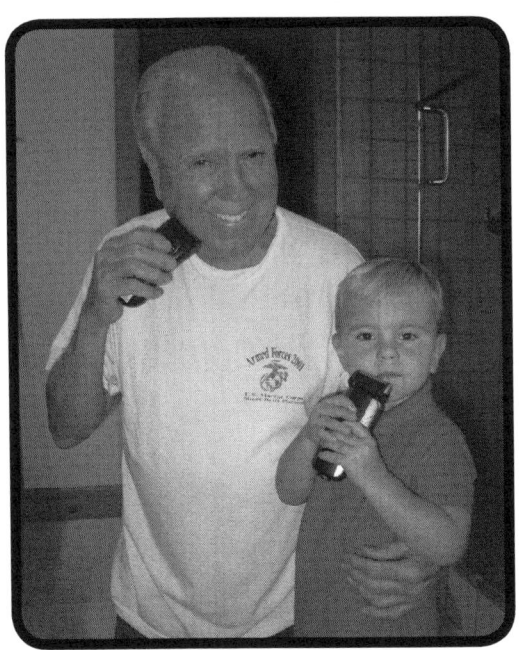

Pictured here with Charlie and my wife Anna at our niece's christening in Madison, New Jersey.

Shaving with Charlie during our normal daily routine. Even something as simple as shaving in the morning would become tedious after my operation.

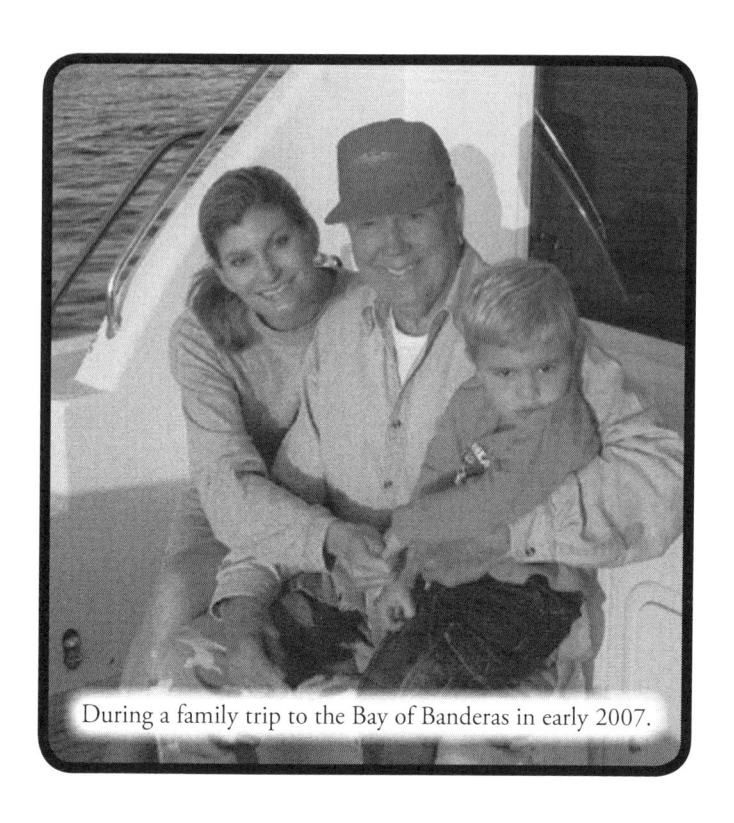

During a family trip to the Bay of Banderas in early 2007.

The fishhook scar on top of my head two days post-operation (the staples were later removed with alligator clips similar to what you would use in an office to remove a staple from a series of joined papers).

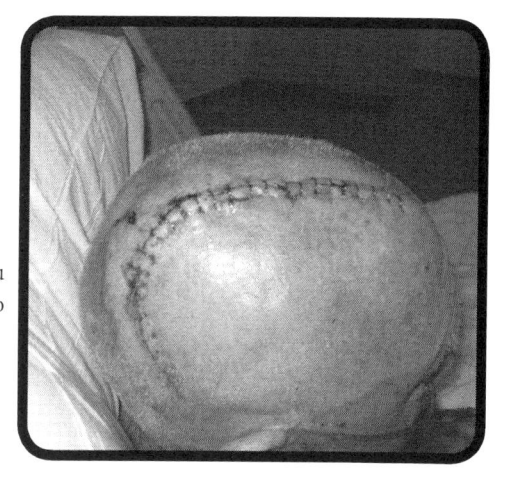

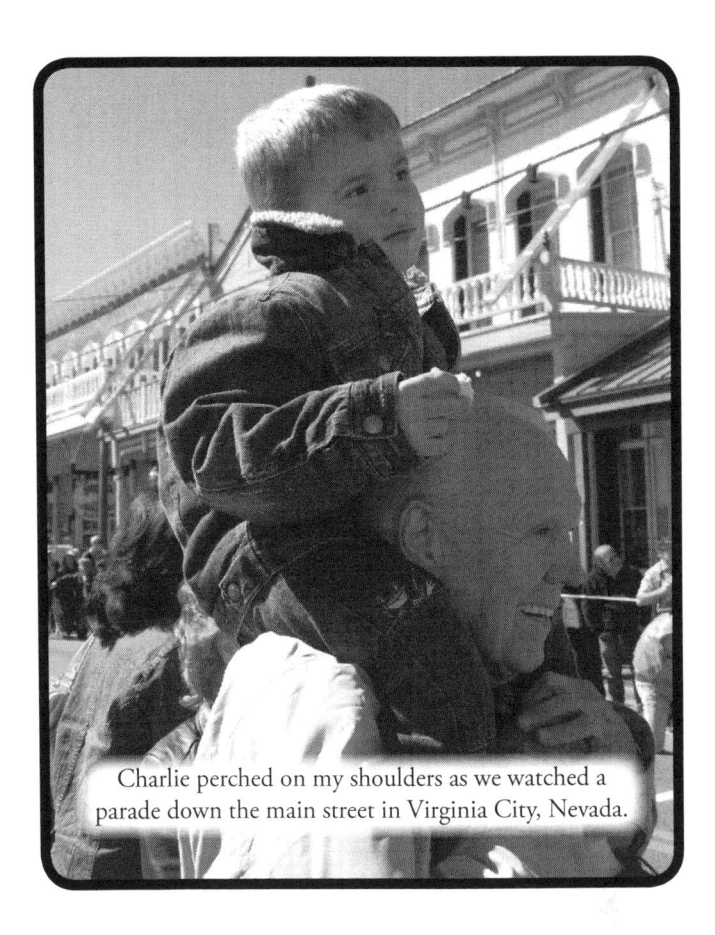

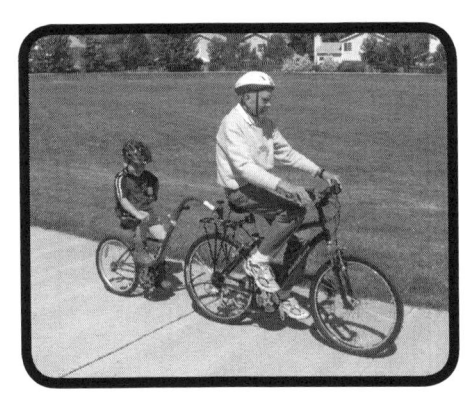

Charlie perched on my shoulders as we watched a parade down the main street in Virginia City, Nevada.

Tandem bicycling with Charlie in a neighborhood park. Pleased to be getting back to father-son activities with Charlie (notice we both have our helmets securely fastened!).

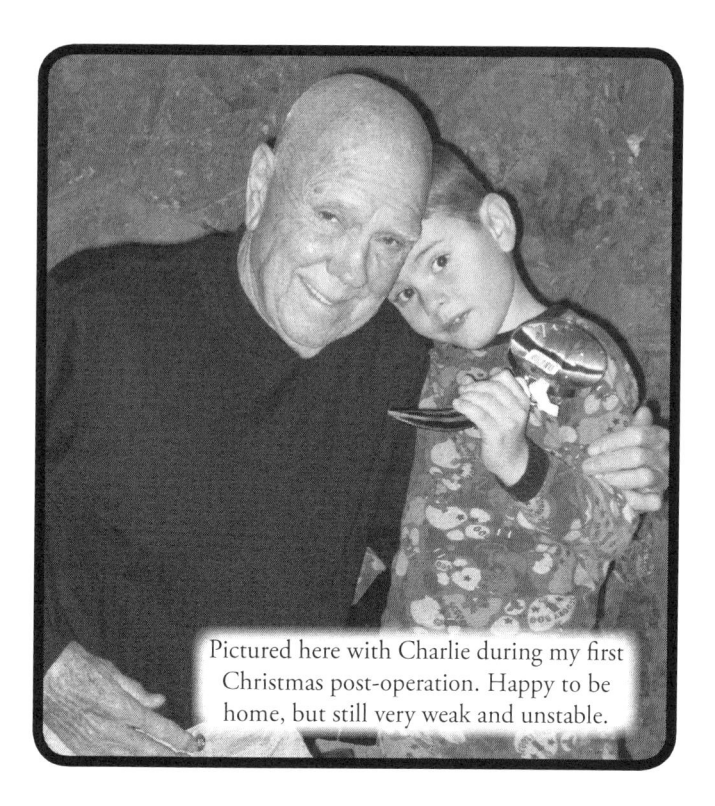

Pictured here with Charlie during my first Christmas post-operation. Happy to be home, but still very weak and unstable.

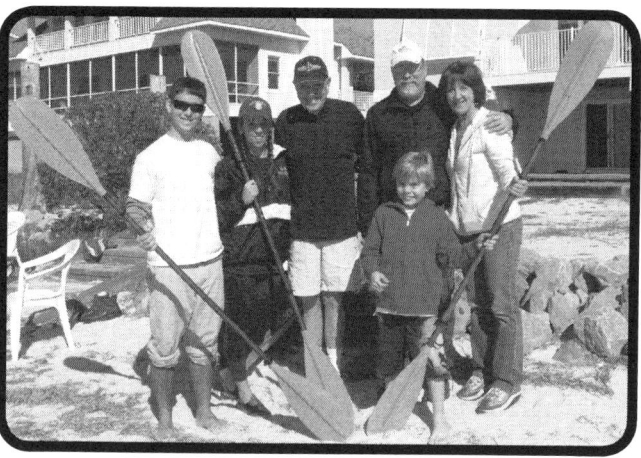

Family gathering at our home in Pensacola, Florida. Pictured here on what we have named "Charlie's Beach" with (from left to right) Doug, Chelsea, Hal Junior, Charlie and Hal Junior's wife Jo.

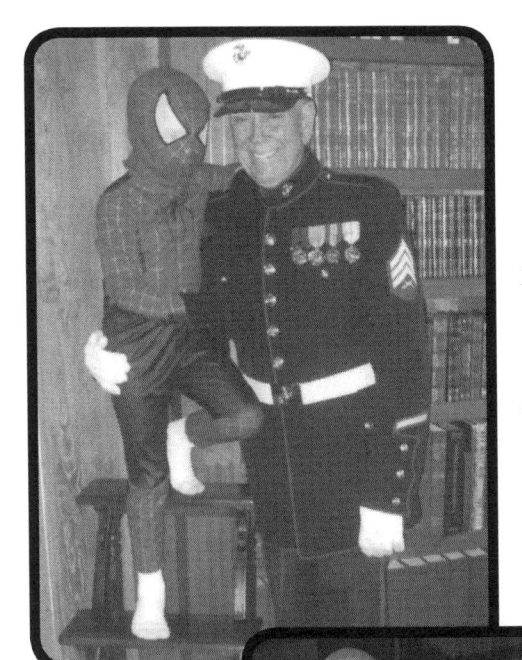

Memorial Day 2009: Another promise fulfilled as I wear my dress blues here with Spiderman (Charlie).

Pictured with my grandson Joseph at his high school graduation.

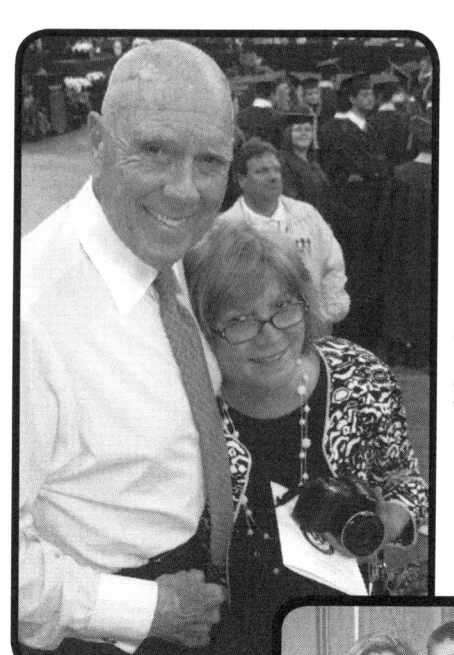

Pictured here with my lovely daughter Debi at my grandson Joseph's high school graduation.

Family photo with our dog Alexander the Great.

Epilogue

Over two and one half years have passed since my skull was put back together and my eyes opened to a life that would be changed forever—a lifestyle that I tried very hard to restore to normal and, in turn, make my brain surgery a non-event. But, in spite of a well above average positive attitude, it was not meant to be. The current overused phrases, "That was then, this is now," and "It is what it is," fit this day's assessment perfectly.

It is hard to put myself into a demographic of tens of thousands of men and women who face annually the life-threatening challenge of a brain injury, stroke and/or any other medical situation requiting the high-risk gamble of brain surgery and follow-up treatment and therapy. The cause, effect and treatment are a one-of-a-kind equation. This is not a team sport. There was no group therapy. The basic instinct to survive kicks in and narrows one's field of interest down to one. When the favorable result of my recovery was beginning to register with me, my concern was to focus towards others less fortunate than I.

The motivation to monitor, record and demonstrate via a book for the benefit of others is a departure from the self-centered helplessness of my earlier state. I am convinced discipline to the mental and physical therapy early in the recovery process not only pays dividends, but also is important to improve the outcome. I too believe attacking the problem with personal dedication as early as possible is a blessing; not capitalizing on this early opportunity is a curse. In my rehab sessions, I could always find someone worse off than I was. I could also spot people that were just going through the motions, putting very little effort into the time-proven methods to help restore the brain and body. Ergo, getting little in return/results. This, in my opinion, postpones a treasured recovery, and in fact, could put it out of reach forever. If you are reading this book because of a personal related interest, either as a patient or someone you know or have a relationship with, it is my wish that in some small way my results and insights might contribute to elevating a recovery to a higher level. When I asked the nurses to "Please leave the lights on," I was working the simplest of functions—one step at a time. To have been able to read a journal of a like-victim's story would have been golden.

The range of emotions I experienced—from the minute Doctor Morgan gave me the bad news rolling me down to the operating room until this very moment—touch every compass point. I never had the luxury of a complete recovery. This, in afterthought, was a mistake. I did not have the dedicated executives willing to fight the economic battles that were brewing (e.g. rogue bankers, an out of control FDIC and an anti-business federal government). A dying owner at worst, a mentally disabled one at best. It was a massive ship jumping. As Coach Bear

Bryant would say, "I need the best I've got on the field."

I was able to conceal certain handicaps relating to my conditions through sheer force of my determination. I would not recommend doing this. I did and still do not have that choice. Nothing excites unethical businessmen more than a weakened opponent, access to unlawful inside information, goal-sharing lawyers, system-beating bankers and partners to share in unlawful gains. There is, to this point, absolutely no consequence for unlawful conduct. Hopeful, with time, by way of an excellent legal team and a fair forum, we will get justice.

I am truly blessed: great family, loyal employees, a small group of outstanding advisors, excellent political support, good recovered health, unimpaired mind and untarnished track record.

Semper Fi,
Hal Holder